Influenza Models

Influenza Models

Prospects for development and use

Proceedings of a working group on
epidemiological models of influenza and
their practical application,
Hemingford Grey, England, 28–30 January 1981

Edited by

PHILIP SELBY

Published for

SANDOZ INSTITUTE FOR HEALTH AND SOCIO-ECONOMIC STUDIES

by

MTP PRESS LIMITED
International Medical Publishers
LANCASTER · BOSTON · THE HAGUE

1982

Cover by Peter Davies

Published in the UK and Europe by
MTP Press Limited
Falcon House
Lancaster, England

British Library Cataloging in Publication Data

Working Group on Epidemiological Models of Influenza and their Practical Application *(1981:Hemingford Grey)* Influenza models. 1. Influenza viruses–Congresses I. Title II. Selby, Philip, *1936–* III. Sandoz Institute for Health and Socio-Economic Studies
616.2'030194 QR201.I6

ISBN 0 85200-459-1

Published in the USA by
MTP Press
A division of Kluwer Boston Inc
190 Old Derby Street
Hingham, MA 02043, USA

Library of Congress Cataloging in Publication Data

Working Group on Epidemiological Models of Influenza and their Practical Application (1981:Hemingford Grey, England) Influenza models.

Includes bibliographical references
1. Influenza–Transmission–Mathematical models. 2. Epidemiology–Mathematical models. 3. Influenza vaccines–Mathematical models. I. Selby, Philip, 1936–. II. Sandoz Institute for Health and Socio-Economic Studies. III. Title. [DNLM: 1. Epidemiologic methods–Congresses. 2. Influenza–Occurrence–Congresses. 3. Models, Biological–Congresses. WC 515 W925i 1981]

RA644.I6W66 1981 614.5'18 82-10057
ISBN 0-85200-459-1 (U.S.)

Typesetting by Speedlith Photo Litho Ltd, Manchester
and printed by Butler & Tanner Ltd., Frome and London

Contents

Preface

Kilbourne (1973) described the student of influenza as "continually looking back over his shoulder and asking 'what happened?', in the hope that understanding of past events will alert him to the catastrophies of the future". Experience suggests the futility of such a hope, since the most predictable feature of influenza is its unpredictability. Nonetheless, the stubborn viability of this hope is strongly affirmed by the many attempts, described and discussed in this volume, to develop a useful and practical representation of influenza virus behavior. I hasten to add, however, that the desired model has yet to be perfected.

The existence and usefulness of animal models of infectious diseases of man are well documented. Reproduction of disease by infecting an experimental animal satisfies the third of Koch's four postulates to establish proof of disease causation by a specific bacterium. Animal models also have been extremely useful in studies of the pathogenesis, immunoprophylaxis, and specific therapy of several important diseases, including (with only modest success) influenza. Development of such a model is simple, at least in concept, and can be achieved by one or only a few scientists.

Somewhat analogous to the animal model of a disease is the experimental model of the behavior of a pathogenic agent in a population. If the disease under study is relatively benign, for example the common cold induced by rhinoviruses, or if a susceptible animal host can be infective for other members of the species by mechanisms similar to those involved in human-to-human transmission, the behavior of the agent in a defined population (human or animal) following its experimental introduction can be observed directly. Such studies have, for example, provided critical proof of the short-range airborne transmission of some agents and the spread of others via contaminated fomites.

Modelling the real-life behavior of a pathogen is obviously far more difficult than modelling of the types mentioned above. Of special interest are agent persistence in, and/or disappearance from, a population; the variation in morbidity and mortality over time (seasonal, secular, and especially epidemic occurrence) and between geographic areas; and the speed and direction of geographic spread. These aspects of behavior reflect the complex interaction of agent and host and the influence of environmental factors, especially population distribution and climate. Further, they can be observed and described thanks to an organized capability for reporting specific morbidity and mortality and for carrying out periodic surveys of antibody prevalence.

Many aspects of the agent-host interaction can be described or inferred from direct observations in the laboratory (by microbiologists) and in the community (by epidemiologists). Important among these are mechanisms of transmission; the minimum infecting dose; the periods of latency (until agent shedding begins) and of infectivity (with shedding at infective levels), which determine the minimum and maximum time between onsets in a continuing chain of infections; the clinical consequences of infection (ratio of clinical to subclinical infections, case fatility); and the degree and duration of post-infection immunity. Knowledge of these aspects of agent-host interaction, plus information about a population (its total size, its composition in terms of families, neighborhoods, other mixing groups such as schools and play groups, and the number and distribution of susceptibles within such groups and by age), constitute the basic information needed to construct a model of the behavior of the agent in a population. Since most of this information is expressed quantitatively as variables rather than as constants, the model becomes relatively complex mathematically and corresponding expertise is required of the model builder. Since a single individual rarely possesses the various types of biological and mathematical expertise required, useful epidemiological modelling requires at least some collaboration. Otherwise, as Fine notes in this volume, "there are often severe relevance and communications problems with such models, due to a tendency for them to be developed and discussed in institutions, in journals, and in a language which divorce them from the biomedical community to which they purport to contribute."

The potential usefulness of epidemiological modelling is enhanced by the impossibility of observing the behavior of an agent in the overall population directly, in sufficient detail, and over enough time to understand the epidemic process, and thereby to predict the occurrence of epidemics. A successful model could be used in making reliable epidemic predictions (regarding time and population), so that control measures could be applied in the most effective way. It could also help in predicting the effectiveness of such measures and in suggesting potential new means of control.

This volume is dedicated to the application of such modelling to influenza, chiefly as caused by type A influenza virus. It begins with an outstanding contribution by Dr Paul Fine, which was prepared as a background paper for advance distribution to the participants. Its purpose was to summarize relevant knowledge concerning influenza, to describe the basic types of models applicable and the principles underlying them, and to review and assess epidemiological modelling as applied to influenza. As a virologist-epidemiologist I admire the conciseness, relevance, and essential completeness of Dr Fine's summary, and the lucidity (for the non-mathematician) of his descriptions of models and their application. This latter characteristic is of particular importance since the relevant biomedical information is, I think, more easily comprehensible than are the necessary mathematical concepts. Dr Fine's contribution should serve as a most helpful introduction to the subject for all readers.

The great and continuing public health importance of influenza abundantly justifies major efforts to understand its epidemiology and bring the disease under control. The 1981 Working Group was constituted on the premise that epidemiological modelling can make an important contribution to these objectives. One might, however, question the appropriateness of influenza as a subject for modelling.

Measles provides an attractive example for model builders. Communicability is high, i.e. non-immunes commonly become infected after exposure by direct contact. Infection usually results in clinically characteristic disease, hence a history of previous measles or non-measles experience is relatively reliable, and the outcome of possible exposure is easily and quite accurately observable. The critical periods of incubation and communicability are well established, and vary within reasonably narrow limits. Finally, since infection confers solid, lifelong immunity, the pool of susceptibles is rapidly depleted during epidemics and replenished only slowly by births and immigration. Thus, reasonably reliable data reflecting the behavior of measles virus in a given population can be obtained in retrospect or prospectively, without laboratory assistance, and used to develop and test the validity of models. The difficulties in modelling stem chiefly from efforts to take into account factors that may affect transmission of the virus in specific, non-homogeneous, free-living populations. These include the physical environment (related to season) and the number, distribution, and behavior of susceptibles in the population.

The fact that some quite satisfactory models have been made in the case of measles might be considered as validating the concept of modelling infectious diseases in general. But influenza undoubtedly presents greater difficulties in this regard than measles. The viruses of measles and influenza belong to different branches (para- and ortho-, respectively) of the myxovirus group. More importantly, there are differences in at least two key aspects of agent-host interaction which make epidemiological modelling inherently more complicated for influenza than for measles. First, while influenza infection does cause "typical" disease, similar disease can also be caused by other agents, and many infections are inapparent or cause atypically mild disease. Thus, the complete discovery and specific recognition of infections require laboratory assistance and are impossible to achieve except in small, defined populations under continuing virological surveillance. Second, post-infection immunity can be considered as solid for no longer than the current influenza season. While a decline over time in resistance to reinfection is typical of other respiratory myxoviruses (parainfluenza and respiratory syncytial viruses), such a decline is effectively but unpredictably enhanced by the changing antigenic character of type A influenza virus.

Since the prediction of epidemics is necessarily based largely on knowledge or estimates of the numbers and distribution of susceptibles, and since susceptibility can only be defined in terms of non-immunity to a forthcoming challenge with a virus of unpredictable antigenic character, it is hardly surprising that the present volume contains no description of a model which is able to predict epidemic occurrence well in advance of a season.

Despite this so far insurmountable limitation, there are several ways in which modelling can help to advance understanding of influenza virus behavior. One is in short-term prediction, after the season has begun, of epidemic occurrence in as yet unaffected areas; this may be based on an analysis of geographic spread in previous epidemic seasons or, as Russian workers claim, on the transmission coefficient calculated for an initial epidemic. Another is in exploring the relative merits of various possible intervention strategies in one or another "typical" population. Perhaps more important are the contributions to an understanding of influenza virus behavior that should result from the recognition of key questions raised in the process of model-building, and the use of even simplistic models to explore "the implications of different sets of assumptions concerning dynamical processes" (as stated by Fine).

I have tried to suggest why reliable or useful epidemiological modelling, especially in influenza, is difficult. The reasons are clearly outlined in Fine's background paper and considerably elaborated upon in the proceedings of the meeting. The volume concludes with a series of recommendations which reflect a consensus of Working Group opinion. These are wide-ranging and urge continuing efforts to better describe specific aspects of influenza virus behavior, to make models now used for influenza more easily available, to apply other existing models to influenza, to attempt further practical applications of existing models, and to stimulate (and seek support for) further work in this area. The concluding, possibly optimistic recommendation is that "a similar workshop be convened in two or three years' time for a detailed examination of the results which will have emerged by then." An obviously desirable first step in this direction would be to commission Dr Fine to update his background paper. This should make it evident whether or not the time to convene a new workshop had arrived.

Reference

Kilbourne, E.D. (1973) *J. infect. Dis., 127,* 478–87.

John P. Fox,
professor emeritus,
department of epidemiology,
University of Washington,
Seattle, Washington

Introduction

In January 1976 the Sandoz Institute organized a working group on pandemic influenza, which met in Rougemont, Switzerland.[a] That group was asked to propose solutions to some key problems in the control of influenza pandemics and epidemics, and to formulate conclusions that could be implemented in follow-up activities. One of its conclusions was as follows:

"As an aid to understanding the epidemic process, and as a tool by which epidemics might be predicted, attempts should be made to build a quantitative, computerized model of an epidemic, with input data including the immune status of the population, weather, seasons, population characteristics, etc."

As a follow-up to this conclusion, we organized in January 1981 a working group on epidemiological models of influenza and their practical application. This second group met in Hemingford Grey, England, in January 1981, and the proceedings are reported in this volume. It was set the following objectives:

(1) to review critically work that has already been done,
(2) to see how models might be developed and used for predicting the behavior of epidemics and the effects of different types of intervention,
(3) to identify and discuss promising directions for future research,
(4) to draw conclusions and make recommendations.

The group included many of the world's leading experts on influenza, mathematical modelling, and the spread of epidemics. Unfortunately we were unable to secure the participation of an expert from the USSR, where much interesting work has recently been reported on the use of models in predicting the spread of influenza epidemics, apparently with considerable success. While the Russian work was discussed by the group, the presence of one of its authors might have been an advantage.

[a] Selby, P., ed. (1976) *Influenza: virus, vaccines, and strategy* (Proceedings of a working group on pandemic influenza, Rougemont, 26–28 January 1976), London and New York: Academic Press.

We would like to thank the distinguished members of our working group for their diligent participation in this endeavor. Special thanks are due to Paul Fine, both for contributing the background paper, which is included in full in these proceedings, and for his valuable assistance in planning the meeting. We are particularly indebted also to David Tyrrell, for his help and encouragement in planning and organizing the meeting, as well as for chairing the crucial final session from which the recommendations emerged. Finally, appreciation is due to Christine Emamzadah for typing the manuscript with her usual efficiency.

Philip Selby,
Sandoz Institute
for Health and Socio-Economic Studies,
Geneva

Background paper

Applications of mathematical models to the epidemiology of influenza: a critique

Paul Fine

ABSTRACT

After introductory sections on the basic epidemiology of influenza, and on the place of mathematical models in epidemiological research, the paper reviews the literature on applications of models to influenza. Several aspects of influenza have been investigated in this way, including: patterns of household outbreaks, shapes of epidemic curves, patterns of geographic spread, implications of population heterogeneity, extent and distribution of influenza-attributable excess mortality, and implications of different immunization strategies. It is argued that more modelling work in each of these areas would be worthwhile. Many valuable techniques have now been developed, but these have not yet been applied sufficiently widely or sufficiently critically to make a major contribution to influenza research. Several specific suggestions are made as to problems and approaches which would be particularly useful for such work in the future.

Analyses of household outbreak data could contribute usefully to the continuing debate over the contagiousness of influenza in different settings and to our understanding of relationships between latent, incubation, and infectious periods. The measles literature contains several models, in particular variants of basic chain binomials, which may be appropriate to these problems. Such analyses should examine the possible role of subclinical infections in influenza. Data on seroconversions within families, in addition to clinical histories, would be especially helpful in this regard.

Studies of epidemic patterns might usefully break away from simple mass-action formulations, in order to investigate such important observed phenomena as seasonal effects, weather effects, and non-unimodal curves. Though epidemic influenza has traditionally attracted most attention, it would be useful to explore the mechanisms of endemicity and virus persistence in non-epidemic periods. This could contribute to our understanding of the genesis of annual epidemics and to our ability to break transmission chains by various means.

Geographic spread models provide a particularly important area for research, as they may provide operationally-useful tools for short-term prediction of epidemic spread. Such tools could be of great importance in planning of control operations. Recent modelling work carried out in the USSR has made impressive claims in this regard, and should be critically examined and repeated in other areas.

A powerful family of models has been developed by Elveback and her colleagues, allowing investigation of the implications of population heterogeneity for the dynamics of spread of infection. These models represent one of the more important recent developments in epidemic theory, with obvious relevance to influenza and many other infectious diseases. Further development of these models, and of means for reducing their demands on computer time, are encouraged. It would be particularly useful to link such modelling to detailed epidemiological studies of actual communities.

Several refinements of traditional excess-mortality models have recently appeared, including both Box-Jenkins time series and multiple regression statistical approaches. Such work is important in the context of continuing debates over the impact of epidemic and non-epidemic influenza, and over the allocation of priorities in influenza control policies.

The heterogeneous-community models of Fox and Elveback have permitted a break from traditional simple concepts of herd immunity to explorations of detailed vaccination strategies within complex populations. The methods have recently been adapted to cost-benefit analyses of influenza vaccination programs. Further developments and field-trial testing of such work are encouraged.

It is concluded that mathematical models have considerable potential for both theoretical and applied research on the epidemiology and control of influenza.

1. Introduction

1.1 Rationale and intent

Influenza is not only a subject of great public health importance, but also an object of intense epidemiological and virological fascination. These characteristics have encouraged major public health campaigns, a large literature, many scientific meetings, and continued public, scientific, and governmental interest as well as concern. However, despite this combined effort, influenza remains incompletely understood, largely unpredicted, and almost totally uncontrolled.

Among many different research approaches which have been applied to influenza, there have been several efforts to use mathematical or computer models in investigations of its epidemiology. Since much of this work has been carried out in isolation from mainstream influenza research and has never been reviewed, it may have contributed less than its potential to our understanding of influenza. At a recent international meeting on influenza control organized by the Sandoz Institute (Working Group on Pandemic Influenza, Rougemont—see Selby, 1976) it was suggested that greater use might be made of mathematical models in studies of influenza. This paper, and the meeting for which it is written, are a response to that suggestion.

The paper attempts to bring together the published mathematical work in a manner which is accessible to those with interests in influenza. It aims to provide a critical review of published applications of mathematical models in studies of the epidemiology and control of influenza. Finally, it attempts to contrast current theory with recent observation, in such a manner as to encourage future attempts to apply the powerful tools of applied mathematics to the important outstanding problems of influenza.

1.2 Background—the nature of influenza

Influenza, "the last great plague", probably has a greater impact upon the public health of developed countries, in terms of morbidity, mortality, and economic disruption, than does any other single infectious disease. But what is it? Before discussing models which purport to describe or analyze influenza, one should have a clear idea of what is being modelled. Indeed, this is an essential (though, unfortunately, sometimes neglected) preliminary to any modelling exercise.

Influenza is the clinical illness associated with infection with members of a well-defined group of RNA-containing myxoviruses. This restricted definition is in marked contrast to the lay application of the terms "flu", "influenza", "grippe", etc. to a heterogeneous collection of illnesses characterized by fever, malaise, and respiratory or even gastro-intestinal symptoms. The restriction is important in pointing to a specific biomedical entity whose nature and behavior are now reasonably well defined, if not fully understood, and which is itself responsible for much, if not most, of the morbidity and mortality which fall under the lay application of the term. What follows is a reasonably orthodox view of the basic epidemiological features of influenza[a] (Beveridge, 1977; Dowdle et al., 1974; Fox and Kilbourne, 1973; Selby, 1976; Stuart-Harris and Schild, 1976).

1.2.1 The viruses

Influenza viruses are widespread in nature, having been isolated from several species of mammals and birds. Two subgroups of these viruses, categorized as Types "A" and "B" on the basis of specific nucleocapsid antigens, are important as human pathogens. By far the greatest interest, and virtually all the modelling work, has focussed upon the Type A viruses. This paper thus concentrates upon these Type A viruses, but recognizes that B-group members are receiving increasing attention as causes of epidemic influenza and of associated diseases such as Reye syndrome (CDC, 1978; Retailliau et al., 1979; WHO, 1980). Virological classification of Type A viruses is intimately related to their epidemiological behavior. The classification is based upon extremely labile surface haemagglutinin (H) and neuraminidase (N) antigens, which undergo periodic major "shifts" (e.g. from H_1 to H_2 to H_3, and from N_1 to N_2, between which strains there is very little cross protection) and more frequent minor "drifts" (identified by minor differences in serological tests).

These different virus "strains" are categorized according to a conventional code indicating their year and place of first isolation. The mechanisms underlying the appearance of, and selection for, these different strains are not fully understood. An abbreviated classification of the major antigenic groups of human Type A influenza viruses is presented in Table 1 (WHO, 1980).

Detailed studies have revealed major differences in the epidemiological behavior of different virus strains, for example an initial tendency for "Asian" H_2N_2 viruses to have highest attack rates in teenage groups, and for "Hong Kong" H_3N_2 viruses to attack less selectively by age. In general, these patterns may be explained in terms of the age distribution of protective antibody in the population at the time the viruses were circulating. There is also some evidence that different virus strains may vary in their virulence or pathogenity. This, too, will have implications for patterns of morbidity and mortality attributable to influenza.

---

[a] It is perhaps a reflection of the importance of influenza, and of the fascinating fundamental problems which it raises, that there are numerous unorthodox views of influenza currently under discussion. Most extreme is the neo-miasma hypothesis of Hoyle and Wickramasinghe (1979), according to which influenza viruses are not transmitted between vertebrates but descend from a galactic "life-cloud". And even seasoned investigators have proposed remarkable variants on the orthodox theme. Hope Simpson (1979) has suggested that the viruses are not transmitted by clinical cases except after a year-long latency period is terminated by some ill-defined stimulus related to the earth's latitude. It is not the purpose of this paper to criticize such hypotheses. Students of influenza have little difficulty in doing so. On the other hand, we may note that the implications of such unorthodox views should be testable using the rigorous logic of mathematical models.

TABLE 1

Abbreviated classification of the major antigenic groups of human Type A influenza viruses

Year of first isolation	*Antigens*		*Comment*
	Haemagglutinin	*Neuraminidase*	
1933	H_1	N_1	First isolated in London by Smith, Andrewes, and Laidlaw. Another isolate by Francis, called "PR-8", has been widely studied. It is possible that this shift type was responsible for the great pandemic of 1918.
1957	H_2	N_2	This "double shift" virus is often called "Asian". It apparently displaced the previous H_1N_1 strains.
1968	H_3	N_2	The "Hong Kong" type. This apparently displaced the H_2N_2 strains.
1976	H_1	N_1	The "Russian" type, similar to the pre-1957 antigenic types. Currently co-circulating worldwide with H_3N_2 viruses. Nucleotide analyses indicate close similarity with 1950 Scandinavian strains (Nakajima et al., 1978).

From WHO (1980)

1.2.2 The course of an infection

Infection of man with influenza viruses generally occurs through the respiratory tract mucosa. If a virus succeeds in establishing itself within a human host, this may lead to periods of infectiousness and/or disease, whose occurrence and timing determine the pattern of influenza in a community. We adhere to conventional definitions in what follows:

(a) *Disease:* Clinical influenza, the disease, must be distinguished from infection *per se* with influenza viruses, as an appreciable proportion of infections are not manifested clinically. As these subclinical or "silent" infections may impart immunity, and may even be responsible for some transmission of virus, they are of importance in determining epidemiological patterns. Several authors have estimated that 20–75 % of influenza virus infections are clinically manifest (Carey et al., 1958; Commission on Acute Respiratory Diseases, 1946; Davis et al., 1970;

Francis et al., 1937; Rickard et al., 1940; Salk et al., 1945). To what extent this varies with virus strains is important, but unclear (e.g. Wright et al., 1980).

(b) *Incubation period:* This is the period from onset of infection to onset of clinical disease (Hope Simpson, 1948). It is best measured in point source outbreaks, when exposure can be attributed to a brief period of time. Observations such as those by Sartwell (1950) and by Moser et al. (1979) indicate that the incubation period of influenza is probably roughly lognormal in distribution, with a range from 24 to 72 hours.

(c) *Duration of disease* (if it occurs): Though not of prime importance for studies of the dynamics of transmission, the duration of clinical disease affects morbidity prevalence and is thus reflected in certain statistics used in epidemiological studies. The duration of uncomplicated influenza ranges from 2 to 7 days (Benenson, 1975).

(d) *Severity and mortality*: The severity and case fatality rate of clinical influenza vary with virus strain and with age and health status of the affected individual (e.g. Houseworth and Langmuir, 1974; Wright et al., 1980). In so far as modelling work relates to actual influenza morbidity or mortality data, this is obviously a factor which must be taken into account.

(e) *Infectiousness*: A period of infectiousness (the shedding of "viable" virus particles) occurs in some if not all infected individuals, and in most if not all diseased individuals. But the period of infectiousness is not synchronous with that of disease, nor with that of infection. Furthermore, the degree of infectiousness is probably associated with the amount of virus shed into the environment, and the manner in which this occurs (i.e. as droplets or droplet nuclei) may vary markedly between individuals. The concept that relatively few individuals (sometimes called "superspreaders") are responsible for much of the transmission of airborne pathogens in a population has been current in the tuberculosis field for many years, and has recently gained increased attention with reference to respiratory viruses (e.g. Hattis et al., 1973). There is experimental evidence for such differences in influenza infections of mice (Schulman and Kilbourne, 1963). The recent report of an outbreak of H_3N_2 influenza among airline passengers may be interpreted in this manner (Moser et al., 1979). A large variance in infectiousness may have important implications for the dynamics of influenza virus transfer.

(f) *Latent period*: This is the period from onset of infection to onset of infectiousness (Hope Simpson, 1948). It is of importance in influenza dynamics, as it determines the minimum serial interval, or period between onset of successive cases in a chain of transmission (see Figure 1). The latent period of influenza is probably close to the incubation period, but may in some cases be slightly shorter, i.e. onset of infectiousness occurs at or before onset of clinical disease (Benenson, 1975).

(g) *Duration of infectiousness* ("Period of communicability"): The duration of virus shedding affects the maximum serial interval between successive cases in a chain of transmission (see Figure 1). It is probably of the order of 3 to 6 days (Baroyan et al., 1977; Benenson, 1975).

(h) *Latency*: The notion of virus "latency" is vague but often discussed. It implies the presence of virus within host cells in some masked state which may require a particular stimulus for induction, or expression, or recovery of recognizable virus. A variety of mechanisms might be involved, including persistence of virus genome either in the host cytoplasm or within the nucleus (the recent discovery of reverse transcriptase has removed a previous theoretical barrier for RNA-containing viruses). That some form of latency may be important in the natural history of influenza viruses has frequently been proposed, but not confirmed (Andrewes, 1951; Hope Simpson, 1979; Mau-Lang, 1979).

1.2.3 The transfer of infection between individuals

The transmission of influenza viruses is manifested as a series or "chain" of infected individuals. The fact that subclinical infections frequently occur means that gaps may appear if clinically diseased individuals are used as markers of successive links in the chain. The use of serological tests to identify subclinical links in a chain of transmission is hampered by the difficulty in deducing a precise time of infection from serological evidence alone. Successive links in a chain are separated in time by the "serial interval" (Hope Simpson, 1948), whose rough limits are: minimum = minimum latent period; maximum = maximum latent period plus maximum duration of infectiousness (see Figure 1). The observed interval is also affected by variations in the incubation period. These time factors are important in the construction and interpretation of models of influenza dynamics.

The measurement of transmission potential is conventionally described in terms of the probability of infection transfer under given circumstances. These measures are typically phrased as secondary attack rates, with subtle numerator and denominator differences dependent upon the situation under study. Remarkable differences occur between estimates of transmission potential, e.g. the very high rate reported by Moser et al. (1979) in contrast to generally low household secondary attack rates reported by many authors (Chin et al., 1960; Davis et al., 1970; Jordan et al., 1958). They may indicate important differences in transmission potential between different virus strains, different infected hosts, or different environmental conditions.

FIGURE 1

Diagram showing the course of successive cases in a chain of transmission, the relationship between the latent and incubation periods, and the serial interval

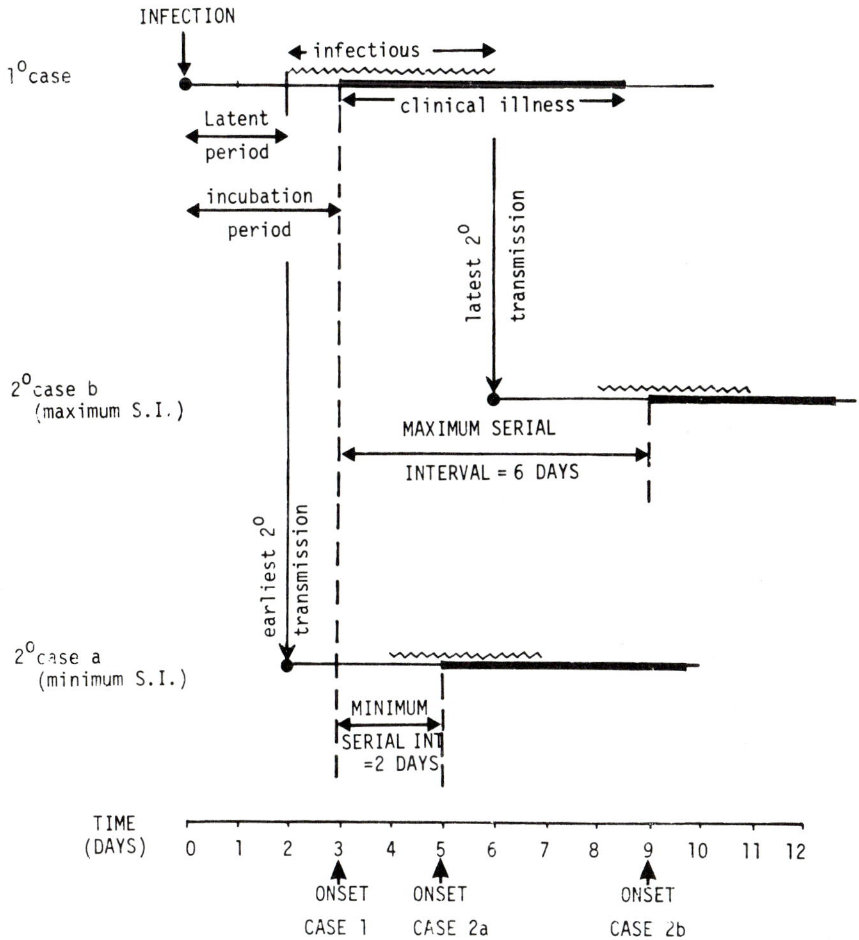

It is assumed for illustration that the latent period is 2 days, the incubation period 3 days, and the duration of infectiousness 4 days. Note that the shortest interval between observed onsets would be 2 days (the latent period), and the longest observed interval would be 6 days (the latent period plus the infectious period).

Influenza viruses are generally carried between individuals through the air in respiratory tract secretions, either within large mucous droplets which travel only a few feet before falling to the ground, or as droplet nuclei (2–4μ in diameter) which may remain suspended in the air for a longer period of time (up to an hour) and be carried for considerable distances (Loosli et al., 1943a,b). The amount of virus shed by infectious individuals, as well as the behavior of these individuals (proximity to other persons, coughing, sneezing, singing, kissing, etc.), probably affects the likelihood of infection transfer. The distribution of these characteristics will determine how uniform is the transmission potential between cases, and may affect the assumptions underlying some models.

Ambient conditions will affect virus viability outside the host, and hence transmission. There is some evidence that low humidity and low temperatures predispose to virus survival and transfer (Hope Simpson, 1958; Loosli et al., 1943b). More subtle factors may also be involved. Schulman and Kilbourne (1963) found that transmission of PR 8 strain influenza virus between mice occurred more readily during winter months than during summer, despite the maintenance of constant temperature and humidity within the laboratory. This finding has not been confirmed. The tendency for influenza to occur during the colder months, both north and south of the equator, has thus led to discussion of a still undefined "winter factor" which predisposes to virus transmission (e.g. Beveridge, 1977).

The confounding of host factors (e.g. crowding in unventilated rooms) and environmental factors (e.g. winter weather) raises important methodological problems for studies of factors associated with virus transmission.

1.2.4 Patterns in space and time

The pattern of influenza within communities has been described in detail in a number of excellent studies (e.g. Carey et al., 1958; Chin et al., 1960; Davis et al., 1970; Dunn et al., 1959; Hope Simpson, 1970; Jordan et al., 1958; Mantle and Tyrrell, 1973; Retailliau et al., 1979; Rickard et al., 1940). Though several of these studies have relied upon data collection through questionnaire, they have provided serological and virological evidence that, at least during known epidemics, people's impressions and memories are reasonably sensitive and specific indicators for clinical influenza.

Influenza frequently strikes communities with a suddenness and explosiveness, in terms of the rapidity with which a large number of persons become involved, which is almost unique among infectious diseases. Attack rates may be very high, but generally differ appreciably between different age and social groups in a population (e.g. the special involvement of high-school students in the H_2N_2 "Asian" epidemic of 1957-58, and the involvement of primary school children with the H_1N_1 "Russian" virus in 1977-78). These differences in attack rates probably reflect differences in specific or cross-reacting immunity levels, and differences in contact patterns, within and between these social groups. Transmission probably occurs wherever people congregate. However, many investigators have found rather low secondary attack rates within families, compared to attack rates in communities as a whole (e.g. Chin et al., 1960; Davis et al., 1970; Hope Simpson, 1979; Jordan et al., 1958). This apparent paradox has encouraged some of the unorthodox views of influenza virus transmission, and provides a nice problem for analyses of infection dynamics within communities.

There are several reports of influenza striking a community in a "second wave", soon after the first (e.g. Chin et al., 1960; Mantle and Tyrrell, 1973). To what extent such recurrences are due to antigenic variants, or to peculiarities in the dynamics of transmission within communities, or to factors such as weather, is unclear.

The broader pattern of influenza is remarkable both for its regularity, which is so tantalizing as to encourage repeated attempts to forecast influenza epidemics, and its irregularity, which has frequently foiled these attempts at prediction.

The temporal pattern is dominated by world-wide "pandemics", which occur at intervals of perhaps 10-40 years and are associated with major shifts in viral H and/or N antigens. These antigenic shifts produce a virus against which a large proportion of the population, and virtually all its younger members, are unprotected. Pandemics may involve very large numbers of individuals, but generally wane after having affected only 30-60% of a population. Between pandemics there are repeated annual epidemics of influenza, involving successive drift variants of previous pandemic strains.

In general, influenza is a seasonal disease, with highest incidence occurring during the colder months, as is typical for many respiratory viruses (e.g. rhinoviruses, measles, mumps). The low incidence of confirmed influenza in summer months has led to hypotheses that the virus enters some latent phase, or even seeks refuge in other species, during the summer. Such hypotheses may not be necessary, however, as increased surveillance has revealed influenza virus activity in northern temperate zone human populations during every month of the year.

It is probable that several seasonal factors related to host physiology, host behavior, and ambient conditions combine to favor virus transfer during winter months and hence the normal winter increase in incidence. Interesting exceptions to the winter epidemics are consistent with this, for example the large outbreak of H_2N_2 Asian influenza in July

1957 in Tangipahoa Parish, Louisiana, a community whose school term begins in June rather than in September (Carey et al., 1958; Dunn et al., 1959). The coincidence of the aggregation of large numbers of susceptible students with the chance arrival of the new double-shift virus, to which the population was highly susceptible, apparently produced conditions for the high transmission rates seen in this epidemic.

On a broader geographic scale, the tendency for influenza incidence to peak in colder months leads to an oscillation of influenza activity between the northern and southern hemispheres, at approximately six-month intervals. This pattern is common to many respiratory viruses. Given the apparent importance of human-to-human transmission in influenza virus maintenance, one might expect influenza activity to follow major paths of travel and population movement. Such a pattern is not always easily demonstrated, however (e.g. Isaacs and Andrewes, 1951),[a] a paradox which has encouraged some of the less orthodox views of influenza virus ecology. It is probable that a collusion of several host and environmental factors underlies the geographic and temporal patterns of influenza activity.

Several of the recent pandemic variants have been first isolated in Asia (H_2N_2 "Asian" in 1957; H_3N_2 "Hong Kong" in 1968; and H_1N_1 "Russian" in 1977), leading to hypotheses that some feature of the overall ecology of Asia might be conducive to whatever mutation, recombination, or interspecies-transfer event may be responsible for the appearance of radically new antigenic types in the population. The possible role of animals in this regard has been discussed ever since it was deduced that the virus responsible for the great 1918 pandemic was similar to a virus endemic in swine in North America (e.g. Shope, 1936). Hypotheses that new antigenic variants arise through genetic recombination of viruses from different host species, or that birds, which carry many influenza viruses, might be important in the world-wide dispersal of influenza viruses, are interesting but not fully confirmed (Beveridge, 1977; Webster et al., 1973).

One of the outstanding features of influenza virus epidemiology is the successive replacement of "old" strains by "new" ones. Until recently it was considered that only one, or very few, virus strains circulated in the human population at one time, and that the displacement of one strain by a successor was rapid over much of the world (e.g. Dowdle et al., 1974).

[a] Dr N. T. J. Bailey tells the author that he has examined the apparent movement of pandemic viruses, as revealed by virus isolation reports, and compared this with statistics on major population movements around the world. The patterns were not strikingly similar. For an alternative view, see the discussion of work by Baroyan, Rvachev, et al. in Sections 2.4.2 and 2.5.1.

This view has changed in recent years, as improved surveillance of influenza viruses has revealed that different drift (and even different shift) strains of virus can circulate simultaneously within countries, communities, and even families (Hope Simpson, 1979; Kendal et al., 1978; WHO, 1979). This recent recognition of co-circulation of influenza viruses demonstrates that we are still learning fundamental properties of the behavior of these viruses, properties which are essential for attempts to model, let alone to control, influenza.

1.3 Background – the nature of models

A model is a simplified representation of an actual process or phenomenon. Its use in biomedical research (animal models, *in vitro* models, computer models, etc.) has obvious advantages and needs no apology. Mathematics and computers provide attractive media for model construction, in terms of flexibility, economy, and relative immunity from ethical constraints. They are especially appropriate for investigation of population problems such as arise in epidemiological studies. On the other hand, mathematical models have the drawback of over-abstraction, a tendency to over-simplify problems to such an extent that the real world may no longer be recognizable in the model. In addition, there are often severe relevance and communications problems with such models, due to a tendency for them to be developed and discussed in institutions, in journals, and in a language which divorces them from the biomedical community to which they purport to contribute.

1.3.1 Types of models

Mathematical models may take a variety of forms. The jargon used to describe these forms is messy, a favorite topic of heated (and generally unproductive) debate by enthusiasts. There follows a lexicon of terms frequently applied in discussions of mathematical, epidemiological models. It should be emphasized that there is considerable overlap between several of these terms.

A posteriori models begin by fitting mathematical expressions to observed data, attempting thereby to induce principles underlying these data. Though applied in infectious disease studies in the early years of this century, this approach has now been generally abandoned in favor of the *a priori* method (Fine, 1979).

A priori models use mathematical logic to explore the implications of sets of assumptions describing the mechanism considered to underlie a phenomenon. The model's predictions may then be compared for consistency with observed data (Fine, 1975; Ross, 1915).

Statistical models are derived from probability theory mathematics, and provide estimates of the probability that certain relationships could hold, or that certain outcomes could arise, by chance, given certain simple underlying relationships.

Descriptive is a term applied to models which aim primarily to describe observed phenomena rather than to mimic the mechanism underlying these observed data. Such models are thus akin to the *a posteriori* or *statistical* models of other terminologies. The phrase *descriptive* models is used by some authors in contrast to *dynamic* models.

Dynamic models aim at a portrayal of the mechanism or process underlying observed phenomena. The term is rather similar to *a priori* as used by earlier authors such as Ross.

Analytical models depend on algebraic manipulation alone in order to explore relationships between variables.

Simulation models depend on numerical substitution and (often repeated or reiterated) solution of algebraic or computer formulations in order to explore their implications.

Discrete time models treat time as divided into successive discrete units of equal duration, typically labelled t, $t+1$, $t+2$, etc. They employ the algebra of finite difference equations, e.g. $S_{t+1} = S_t - C_{t+1}$ means the number of susceptibles in the next time period (S_{t+1}) equals the number susceptible in this time period (S_t) minus the number of cases in the next time period (C_{t+1}).

Continuous time models treat time as a continuous variable, and employ the differential calculus to specify rates of change at points in time. Thus $dy/dt = \beta xy$ means that the rate of change of the prevalence (y) with time is equal to the product of the number of susceptibles (x) times the number of cases (y) times a transmission factor β.

Deterministic models allow no variation due to chance, and hence provide only a single solution or prediction for any given formulation and set of initial conditions.

Stochastic models include a chance function, and thus their results are expressed in terms of probabilities, or probability distributions, of possible outcomes. Some simple stochastic models are analytical, but most depend on computer simulation for their solution.

1.3.2 Uses of models

Insofar as mathematical modelling may be carried out in isolation from subject matter disciplines, it may justify itself in terms of contributions to mathematics or to computer science alone. In this paper, however, we restrict our interest to the potential contribution of models to our understanding of the epidemiology of, and our ability to control, influenza. There are at least six ways in which models may contribute to epidemiology and public health.

First, models may provide useful tools for the *description* of observed data. Many statistical models are of this sort, as are the time series analyses applied to influenza mortality data, or the so-called "catalytic models" for age prevalence data (Muench, 1959).

Second, models are useful in allowing *exploration* of the implications of different sets of assumptions concerning dynamic processes.

Third, models are useful in *hypothesis testing*. Indeed, a model may be considered as a rigorous formulation of a complex hypothesis whose validity may be tested by the comparison of its predictions with reality.

Fourth, models may be useful in *prediction* of future events, and hence as operational guides for control programs. Though many models are currently used in guiding decisions concerning physical systems (e.g. power circuits) and even in economics (though with questionable results·), there are few examples of models being used in public health decision-making. It is important in the context of this review that some influenza models may come closer to operational uses than do models of any other infectious diseases.

Fifth, models play an important role in the *teaching* of epidemiological principles in some schools of public health. Indeed, it is by making students aware of the subtleties of the dynamics of infectious processes that models have probably had their greatest impact on the actual practice of public health.

Sixth, the very *process of model building* is undoubtedly useful because of the questions it raises and the logical demands it entails. Anyone who has ever "built" a model is aware of this. For this reason alone, model building deserves a place as part of a research exercise.

A word of caution is necessary here. It is easy to be too facile in speaking of the usefulness of models. An enterprise cannot survive on potential alone, and one may well question to what extent the large literature on mathematical epidemiological models has lived up to any potential usefulness. It is probably correct to say that it has not—though it is also probably correct to say that this potential has sometimes been over-rated by enthusiastic partisans. Among the major reasons for the failure of modelling to have a greater practical impact are those of difficulties in communication, discussion in isolation, and lack of self-criticism. This paper attempts to address some of these deficits.

Finally, it is important to note a rather special problem related to the usefulness of mathematical models. Their very elegance may beguile—especially in the face of the bewildering complexities of the real world. What is more, they may beguile so much as to mislead. Thus Langmuir, one of the foremost public health officers of this century, and himself sympathetic to the use of models in epidemiological investigations, has questioned whether simplistic models may have misled a generation of public health workers into too naive a view of herd immunity (Langmuir, 1977). And Armitage, one of the foremost contemporary medical statisticians, has warned that, in dealing with models, "we should be wary of 'insight' which is separated by a thin dividing line from self deception" (Armitage, 1975). This is wise advice.

2. Review and commentary

2.1 Introduction

This section presents a review of published work relating to the application of mathematical models to influenza. A literature search has uncovered approximately 50 such publications, all of which are cited in the bibliography. I have been unable to obtain copies or translations of several papers, which I have thus not actually read. These unconsulted references are indicated by asterisks.

It is probable that discussions of great relevance to influenza are to be found in publications not directly aimed at models of influenza. On the other hand, it is not possible to review the complete mathematical epidemiology literature here, and therefore it has been necessary to set boundaries regarding both subject matter and methodology for the studies included in this review. Thus references are made to work on the common cold, a disease complex whose ecology bears some similarities to that of influenza. Several studies of measles are also mentioned, not only because this infection shares certain important epidemiological similarities with influenza, but also because of the extent and quality of the published work on measles. With regard to methodology, the boundaries have been drawn so as to include some work which might be described as statistical data analysis, rather than modelling. This is particularly true with reference to the work on excess mortality. The boundaries between model building and statistical analysis are not clearly defined, however, and it has been considered that more is to be gained by inclusion than by exclusion of disputed territory.

Rather than discuss each paper separately, or order them according to mathematical form, it has been considered preferable to treat them in groups according to the aspect, or "level", of influenza epidemiology to which they refer: i.e. family or transmission studies; small community studies; large population studies; prediction and control studies. An effort is made to emphasize both the epidemiological and the modelling features of the studies, with reference to the general principles outlined in the previous section.

Algebra has been de-emphasized, and largely banished to an appendix. An effort is made to describe the mathematical arguments and results in words alone. Hopefully this will attract that most important group of readers who are seriously interested in and knowledgeable about influenza, and who have decision-making powers regarding influenza control, but who are put off by pages of mathematical symbols.

A little algebra has been unavoidable. In presenting this, I have applied a consistent set of symbols throughout (see Glossary). This has inevitably meant changing the symbols used by many original authors—but the alternative would have been hopelessly confusing. To simplify matters further, the symbol S means susceptible, and C a case.

2.1.1 Paradigms of contagion

The epidemiology of influenza depends upon the transmission of virus between infected and susceptible individuals. It is important to consider how this fundamental process is included in models which attempt to describe the dynamics and patterns of the disease. A survey of the literature reveals that most authors have employed one of two classical approaches to this problem, either the "mass action" or the "Reed-Frost" formulation.

The epidemiological "mass action" principle was proposed first by William Hamer, in 1906. The concept was later elaborated by Ross (e.g. 1915), by Soper (1929), and by Kermack and McKendrick (1927), the latter authors being most frequently cited in the modern literature. It may be simply stated thus:

The incidence (rate) of new cases of infection is a function of the product of the number of current cases times the number of current susceptibles.

Hamer phrased this in simple discrete form, as:

$$C_{t+1} = S_t \cdot C_t \cdot b \qquad (1)$$

where C_t, C_{t+1} = numbers of cases (infected and infectious individuals) at times t and $(t+1)$ respectively. The time interval is taken as the serial interval of the infection in question, and a case is considered infectious during a single time period.

S_t = number of susceptibles at time t.

b = a transmission coefficient, given different names by different authors. It represents the proportion of all possible contacts between susceptibles and cases, in one time period, which lead to new infections.

Hamer implicitly recognized that the *b* is a reciprocal of the "epidemic threshold", i.e. the number of susceptibles which, if exceeded, will lead to an epidemic (increase in incidence). This relationship, which may have important theoretical implications for influenza and its control, is elaborated in Appendix A.

The continuous time versions of the mass action principle are generally phrased as:

$$\frac{dy}{dt} = x \cdot y \cdot \beta \tag{2}$$

where x = number of susceptibles

y = number of infectious cases

β = "transmission rate" (called by different names)

$\frac{dy}{dt}$ = "derivative of y with respect to t", i.e. the rate of change in y with time.

Whereas the discrete time mass action model of Hamer assumed that a case is infectious for one time period, and then recovers, the continuous time models generally assume that cases recover at a constant rate (see Appendix B).

The mass action principle is easily manipulated algebraically, and it provides predictions of epidemic curves which resemble some observed data. It is the most widely used description of infectious processes in the epidemiological modelling literature. It is not without failings, however. One problem is its implicit assumption of random mixing. This assumption is often made in mathematical models, for the sake of tractability, but it can be misleading when models are applied to actual populations. Methods to avoid this assumption are discussed in Section 2.3.2. A second problem with the mass action formulations is the meaning of the transmission coefficients *b* or β.[a] Their relationship to theoretical epidemic thresholds is interesting; but they do not have meanings which allow their direct measurement in epidemiological studies. A third problem with the mass action model is its implicit

[a] The *b* and β parameters of the discrete and continuous mass action models, respectively, have been called "transmission coefficients", "transmission rates", "contact rates", "forces of infection", "transmissibility factors", "infection rates", even "infectivity", by different authors. This is unfortunate, especially as several of these terms evoke biological concepts which are much better described by other parameters (such as conventional secondary attack rates or the Reed-Frost "probability of effective contact" as discussed below). It is probable that the confusion engendered by this semantic morass has had a detrimental impact on the development of infectious disease epidemiology (see Fine, 1979).

assumption that, if the number of susceptibles were kept constant, then the incidence (rate) would vary linearly with the prevalence of infectious cases (i.e. $C_{t+1}/S_t = C_t \cdot b$). In the discrete time formulation this can lead to an absurd prediction of more new cases than there are susceptibles – in other words, a combination of high C_t and b values can suggest $C_{t+1} > S_t$. This problem does not arise if the number of cases is very small in relation to the number of susceptibles (in which situation few susceptibles would contact more than one case), but it does make the mass action equation inappropriate for studies of small populations.

Two of the three main problems underlying the mass action model are resolved in a model derived by Lowell Reed and Wade Hampton Frost in the late 1920s (Abbey, 1952; Fine, 1977; Frost, 1976). Though the assumption of random mixing is still employed, the transmission of infection is now defined in terms of a probability p = "probability of effective contact" = the probability that any two individuals in the population have, during one time interval (the serial interval of the infection in question), that sort of contact which is necessary for infection transfer. Indeed, p is just the conventional secondary rate subsequent to a single primary case: i.e. the number of cases to arise between 1 minimum and 1 maximum incubation period after exposure to the primary case, divided by the total number of susceptibles exposed to the primary case. And the basic model is:

$$C_{t+1} = S_t\{1 - (1 - p)^{C_t}\} \tag{3}$$

or

$$C_{t+1}/S_t = 1 - (1 - p)^{C_t} \tag{4}$$

i.e. the incidence (rate) in the next time period is that number (proportion) of susceptibles who make "effective contact" with *at least one* case in the current time period. The derivation is clarified in Appendix C. Algebraically, the Reed-Frost expression is somewhat more clumsy than is the mass action, and this has discouraged its wide use in epidemiological theory. On the other hand, this difficulty has been overcome by using computer simulation, thus allowing full benefit of the assumptions underlying the model.

We will meet both the mass action and the Reed-Frost expressions repeatedly in the pages which follow, in the context of specific influenza models. One general comparative comment about the two models may not be inappropriate at this stage. It is of interest that the mass action expression is used almost universally by workers with a mathematical background; whereas those with epidemiological backgrounds seem more liable to favour the Reed-Frost formulation. Certainly the Reed-Frost model provides the more reasonable description of small populations or of conditions where the contact or transmission rate is high. On the other hand, it can be shown that the two models are virtually identical when applied to conditions where the probability of effective contact is very low (see Appendix D).

2.2 Models of influenza in families

Families provide particularly useful subjects for epidemiological studies. They present well-defined groups of individuals who share similar environments, and about whom information may be relatively easily gathered. It is often possible to obtain reasonably accurate clinical information on all members of a family through a single cooperative informant. The intimacy of contact between family members encourages transfer of contagious infections, and provides good opportunities to study the relationship between successive cases in a chain of transmission.

Several models have been developed which are particularly relevant to family data. These have been applied to a limited extent to influenza, in order to investigate questions such as the following:

(1) Is there clear evidence of person-to-person transmission of influenza within families?

(2) What is the time relationship between successive family cases, in terms of latent period, incubation period, and duration of infectiousness?

(3) What is the risk of influenza transmission between family members?

To these three questions should be added a fourth, which is of great potential interest and to which family studies are especially appropriate:

(4) What are the differences in the behavior of different influenza viruses within similar families, or in the behavior of the same virus within different families?

Household data provide series of cases, by date of onset. The first problem in their analysis is that of deducing the relationship between the cases. The simplest approach has been to call all cases "secondaries" which arise during some arbitrary interval following onset of the index case (e.g. within 10 days, as in Davis et al., 1970) or between 1 minimum and 1 maximum incubation period after onset of the first case. Hope Simpson (1948) recognized that the interval between primary and secondary cases, i.e. the serial interval, is determined more by the latent period than the incubation period, and is best determined by analyzing the frequency distribution of intervals between onsets of family cases.

Bailey then developed a statistical model which provides estimates of the mean and standard deviation of the latent period (assumed normally distributed), the duration of the infectious period (assumed constant), as well as the intra-familial transmission rate, from data on the time distribution between cases in families. Bailey (1975) describes the model and its application to measles data, for which it provides reasonable estimates of these important parameters. Owada et al. (1971) applied the model to data on influenza B within 1,022 families in Osaka, deriving an estimate of 4.7 days as a mean latent period and 2 days as the effective duration of infectiousness. Though not unreasonable, this latent period appears rather long, and the infectious period rather short, at least in comparison with estimates for influenza A by several other workers (Davis et al., 1970; Elveback et al., 1976; Moser et al., 1979; etc.). One may wonder whether this is a valid reflection of influenza B behavior in this population, or whether data inaccuracies, missed subclinical cases, or late co-primary cases (i.e. contracted outside the families) could have affected the result. These are questions of great interest in influenza, as a valid identification of successive links in a transmission chain is an essential preliminary to estimating transmission factors, and in calculating intervals, durations, and rates.

The models most often applied in studies of intra-familial contagion are the so-called "chain binomials", of which the Reed-Frost is a special case. These discrete models consider the courses of intra-familial mini-epidemics as series of binomial trials, each exposed susceptible having a certain probability of becoming infected at each successive "generation" of cases. For the classic chain binomial model of Greenwood (1931), each susceptible in the family has a constant probability p^* of becoming infected, in each serial interval. For the Reed-Frost, this probability changes, being $1 - (1 - p)^{C_t}$ in each interval, where C_t is the number of cases to which each susceptible is exposed during that interval (see Appendix C). Note that these probabilities are identical for situations in which there is but a single source case (i.e. if $C_t = 1$). It is also relevant to note that the p in the Reed-Frost is identical to the conventional secondary attack rate subsequent to a single primary case, whereas the chain binomial p^* is similar to Hope Simpson's (1952) "susceptible exposure attack rate". Despite the fact that the Reed-Frost model has greater intuitive appeal, as it takes into account the number of potential source cases present in each interval within a family, the simple chain binomial has received greater attention in the literature, probably because of its greater mathematical tractability. Bailey (1975) reviews the literature on both models, with emphasis on methods for obtaining best estimates of p^*, or p, the transmission parameters, from sets of family data (Appendix E).

Development of chain binomial theory has taken place largely with reference to measles, for which there are several carefully collected data sets available. After Greenwood (1931) found good agreement between the distribution of total numbers affected in families and the chain binomial predictions, Wilson et al. (1939) pointed out that the model did not fit data broken down into actual chains of 1°, 2°, 3°, etc. cases. In particular, too many secondary cases were observed, relative to tertiary cases. There followed a series of discussions by Greenwood (1949), Bailey (1953, 1956 – reviewed in Bailey, 1975), and Ipsen (1959), each developing variants to the basic chain binomial in order to investigate whether the peculiarities of measles data were explicable in terms of variation in transmission between households or within them (e.g. related to age difference between cases and susceptibles).

Both Greenwood chain binomial and Reed-Frost models have been applied to household common cold data, with interesting results. Thus Heasman and Reid (1961) estimated effective contact rates (Reed-Frost p) of 0.12 in crowded households, which was insignificantly higher than the 0.10 value found for uncrowded households. They further noted an improved fit using Bailey's model based on a variable latent and constant infectious period. And Lidwell and Somerville (1951) used these models in studies which revealed a decreased susceptibility (decreased p value) to household common cold transmission with age of the exposed individuals.

Such models have been applied to influenza at least twice. Hope Simpson and Sutherland (1954) applied chain binomials to influenza data collected in Gloucestershire families during the late 1940s, and concluded there was only marginal evidence for transmission within the households. Sugiyama (1960, 1961; see also Yamamoto, 1959) extended the classical chain binomial to include extra- as well as intra-family transmission, and applied this to data on Asian H_2N_2 influenza in Osaka, thereby estimating the risk of intra-household transmission as $p_i^* = 0.23$, compared to an extra-household transmission risk as $p_e^* = 0.04$. These seem to be reasonable estimates, at least in the absence of further information on the epidemiological situation; and the simultaneous consideration of infection sources outside, as well as inside, the family is a useful contribution.

2.3 Models of influenza in small communities

The study of contagious infections in groups of 50 to 5,000 people has several advantages. It allows detailed investigation of epidemiological patterns in actual communities. If an investigation is well planned, communities in this size range can be completely enumerated, characteristics of individuals can be identified in considerable detail, susceptibility of all individuals can be assessed (either by history or serology), case ascertainment can be high, and detailed contact tracing may even allow linkage of successive cases in chains of transmission. There is considerable scope for the application of models to such data, though rather few published examples of such applications which are relevant to influenza.

Such small community modelling investigations are appropriate to answer questions such as the following:

(1) What is the pattern of epidemics in single communities, and how can this pattern be explained in terms of simple factors such as level of immunity in populations, duration and degree of infectiousness, etc.?

(2) How much variation is there in epidemic patterns between similar communities?

(3) What is the relationship between size, population density, social structure, etc. of a community to overall or to detailed epidemic patterns?

2.3.1 Homogeneous community–random mixing models

Most epidemiological models are based upon assumptions of homogeneous, random mixing populations–i.e. susceptibility is uniform between individuals and all susceptibles are equally likely to "contact" cases during any time period. Though such an assumption does not fit comfortably with the well-recognized highly-structured nature of human communities, the assumption is often rationalized as being essential for certain mathematical purposes, and hopefully not too misleading.

The simple discrete time mass action model (Appendix A) has been discussed with reference to influenza by Fortmann and Florin (1975), by Fortmann (1976), and by Damms et al. (1976), though with little reference to actual data. More interesting is the investigation by Hammond and Tyrrell (1971), who applied continuous time mass action theory to data on nine common cold epidemics in the small island population of Tristan da Cunha (less than 300 people). They attempted to fit the basic Kermack-McKendrick equations (Appendix B) to epidemic curve data, estimating the three essential parameters (initial number of susceptibles, contact rate, and recovery rate) by a least-squares method.[a] They found a consistently poor fit between model prediction and actual data, which they attributed to the model's assumption of too high a recovery rate in the early phases of the

[a] This is a standard technique for fitting models to data, by minimizing the sum of the squares of the differences between pairs of observed and expected values.

epidemics (note that the Kermack-McKendrick equations postulate a constant daily recovery rate for all cases). Hammond and Tyrrell then explored an alternative assumption, that cases last for a constant duration D. They found this adaptation of the model led to a rather better fit than did the original. Hammond and Tyrrell also comment on the threshold phenomenon, that epidemics occurred only if the initial number of susceptibles exceeded $1/\beta D$. This of course is inherent in the model, in the definition of β, as their constant duration parameter D is directly analogous to the reciprocal of the recovery rate (i.e. $1/\gamma$) in the Kermack-McKendrick formulation (Appendix B).

The basic Reed-Frost model (Appendix C) has also been fitted to small community epidemic data. The classic study is that of Helen Abbey (1952) who fitted the simple, discrete-time, deterministic Reed-Frost equation to data on outbreaks of measles, chickenpox, and rubella. Her discussion is especially useful because of its critical consideration of the problem of over-estimating susceptibles through false negative histories.

2.3.2 Heterogeneous community–non-random mixing models

Human communities are not homogeneous. Human activities are not random. The contrast between these simple truths and the assumptions of most epidemiological models has concerned all of the more critical students of epidemic theory. These assumptions are especially worrying in the context of influenza studies; for it is well known that influenza attacks, and moves, selectively through communities—an obvious example being the dominant role of teenagers in the pattern of H_2N_2 (Asian) influenza. But only one group of researchers has tackled this problem directly: Fox, Elveback, Ackerman, and their colleagues have produced a major series of publications over the past 15 years, and brought forward results of considerable practical as well as theoretical importance. Several of their papers relate directly to influenza.

This series of publications has entailed a progressive adaptation of the Reed-Frost model to provide increasingly realistic, if complex, descriptions of community epidemics of infectious disease. Because of the complexity of the underlying assumptions, the models have relied on computer simulation, rather than algebraic analysis. The models are fully stochastic. In order to allow for unique characteristics of each member of the study population, at each time period a random device determines whether each individual becomes infected, becomes infectious, recovers, etc. The main characteristics of the seven models thus far produced are outlined in Table 2. Though any of the models could be applied to influenza, Model VII was designed with particular reference to comparative studies of H_2N_2 (Asian) and H_3N_2 (Hong Kong) influenza.

TABLE 2

Summary of Reed-Frost type stochastic simulation models published by Elveback and co-workers

Model number	*Population structure*	*Length of periods*		*Vaccination schedule*	*Reference*
		Latent	*Infectious*		
I	Unstructured, random mixing	Constant	Constant	None	Abbey, 1952
II	,,	,,	,,	None (but viral interference)	Elveback et al., 1964
III	,,	,,	Random variable	Any	Elveback et al., 1968
IV	Structured	,,	,,	,,	Elveback et al., 1971
V	,,	,,	,,	,,	Elveback et al., 1971
VI	Highly structured (pseudo-sociological)	,,	,,	,,	Ewy et al., 1972
VII	Structured	Random variable	,, also variable infectiousness and proportion diseased	,,	Elveback et al., 1975, 1976

Roman numeral designations are those used by the original authors. Model V differs from Model IV in including environmental contamination as well as contact transmission. Model VII was designed with special reference to influenza.

A model population of 1,000 individuals was designed to mimic an American community consisting of 140 pre-school age children, 320 school age children and adolescents, 316 young adults, and 224 older adults. The characteristics of each of these individuals, including "membership" in certain social groups, is coded on separate input cards. Thus there are 30 "play groups" for pre-school age children, each with 2 to 6 members; and neighborhood and social mixing groups are represented by 50 clusters, each containing 3 to 6 different families, etc.

The structure is therefore highly specific, as in a real community. An especially important point is that all the social group assignments in the model are flexible, and any conceivable structuring of the community may be achieved merely by altering the age or social group assignments as coded on the individuals' input cards.

The model keeps track of the status (susceptible, infected but not yet infectious, infectious-diseased, infectious-not diseased, diseased-withdrawn to home, or recovered-immune) of each individual on a daily basis.

The decision as to whether a susceptible individual becomes infected on any day is based on chance. The *probability* that an individual becomes infected, on each day, is calculated on the basis of his or her opportunities for contacting infectious cases within each of his or her different social mixing groups. Probabilities of contact *within* any group are estimated on the basis of the number of infectious cases present, using the basic Reed-Frost equation (Appendix C). Contact probabilities within each group were determined on the basis of attack rates and secondary attack rates as derived in published studies of actual epidemics and on the basis of their implications in simulated epidemics. The values used in simulations of H_2N_2 and H_3N_2 influenza are given in Table 3. The method of calculating the probability of infection for an individual may be illustrated by considering a young adult, "George", during the H_2N_2 epidemic. Say George belongs to a neighborhood cluster which contains, on the day in question, 2 infectious cases. Say there are no cases in George's family on this day, but there are 50 cases in the community at large. Then:

$$\text{Probability}\left\{\begin{array}{l}\text{George is}\\ \text{infected}\\ \text{during day}\end{array}\right\} = 1 - \text{Probability}\left\{\left[\begin{array}{l}\text{George is not}\\ \text{infected in}\\ \text{cluster}\end{array}\right] \text{ and } \left[\begin{array}{l}\text{George is not}\\ \text{infected in}\\ \text{family}\end{array}\right] \text{ and } \left[\begin{array}{l}\text{George is not}\\ \text{infected in}\\ \text{community}\end{array}\right]\right\}$$

$$= 1 - \{(1 - 0.005)^2 (1 - 0.2)^0 (1 - 0.00025)^{50}\}$$

$$= 1 - 0.97773$$

$$= 0.02227$$

The *probability* that George becomes *infected* on the day in question is thus 0.02227.[a] In order to decide whether he *actually* becomes infected,

[a] For computational reasons, the model calculates these probabilities in a slightly different fashion, making use of the fact that $(1 - p)^C \approx e^{-pC}$, if p is small (see Elveback et al., 1975).

TABLE 3

Within-group contact rates ("probabilities of effective contact, per day") used by Elveback et al. (1976) in simulating Asian (H_2N_3) and Hong Kong (H_3N_2) influenza patterns in a community of 1,000

	Children		*Adults*	
	Pre-school	*School*	*Young*	*Older*
Asian H_2N_2				
Family	0.02	0.02	0.02	0.02
Play groups	0.10	—	—	—
Cluster	0.005	0.005	0.005	0.005
School days 1-5	—	0.009	—	—
later	—	0.006	—	—
Total community	0.00025	0.000125	0.00025	0.000125
Hong Kong H_3N_2				
Family	0.02	0.02	0.02	0.02
Play groups	0.05	—	—	—
Cluster	0.009	0.006	0.01	0.009
School	—	0.0015	—	—
Total community	0.00028	0.00026	0.00038	0.00035

Each of these figures reflects the probability that two individuals, in the specified social group, would have "contact" appropriate for transmission of the virus in question, in one day.

the computer is asked to produce a random number uniformly distributed between 0 and 1. If this number turns out to be between 0 and 0.02227, George is considered to have been infected; but if the number is between 0.02227 and 1, George escapes infection on that day.[b]

Once infected, George's subsequent course is also determined to an important degree by chance. Thus the latent and infectious periods are not constants, but are given frequency distributions according to current understanding of influenza.

The latent (pre-infectious) period for the H_2N_2 (Asian) influenza model has the following distribution: 1 day (30%), 2 days (50%), 3 days (20%). A new random number (between 0 and 1) determines whether George's latent period is 1, 2, or 3 days: if the number is between 0 and 0.3, his latent period is 1 day; if the number is between 0.3 and 0.8, it is 2 days; if it is between 0.8 and 1 the period is 3 days. A similar procedure is employed to decide whether the duration of infectiousness is 3 days (30%), 4 days (40%), 5 days (20%), or 6 days (10%). Whether George has clinical

[b] This method for introducing chance in computer models is often called "Monte Carlo".

illness or subclinical infection, and if clinical, whether he is withdrawn (bed rest at home), are similarly decided.

The model works by taking any pre-assigned population and influenza introduction, carrying out the required calculations for each individual on each day, and keeping track of the course of the entire epidemic phenomenon. Being fully stochastic, with each crucial event dependent upon an independent random number, each simulated epidemic will differ in its course. The results of the model are thus presented as means or as frequency distributions of epidemic sizes (or durations or group specific attack rates) predicted by a given set of initial conditions (e.g. Figure 2). In theory, these frequency distributions should resemble the distributions of results of influenza outbreaks in a group of communities similar to the model population. Other output includes distributions of daily epidemic course, and group-specific attack rates of

FIGURE 2

Frequency distributions of total size (total numbers of cases) in 500 simulated Asian epidemics and 200 simulated Hong Kong influenza epidemics

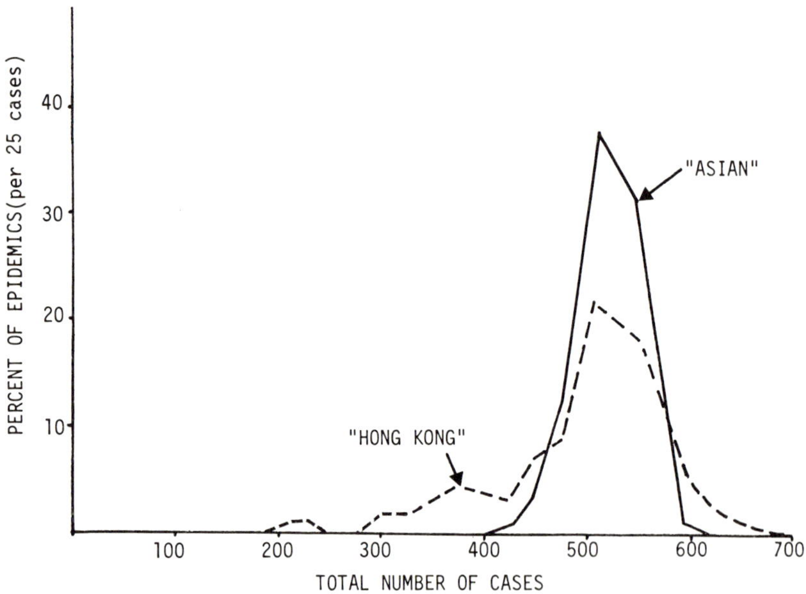

Epidemics simulated in structured populations of 1,000, using parameter values described in the text and in Table 3 (from Elveback et al., 1976a).

infection and of clinical illness. Such model results encourage the testing of detailed hypotheses as to the behavior of influenza in human communities. Their important implications for optimization of control strategies are discussed in Section 2.5.2.

This is clearly a powerful modelling technique. In principle it allows an investigator to come as close as he or she wishes to a representation of the actual details of an epidemiological situation. Any detail which can be specified (formulated in unambiguous terms) can be simulated. It is thus the logical riposte to the model critic who would dispose of models because they do not take this or that detail into account. A particularly nice example of this potential is the adaptation of this model to explore the implications of "superspreaders" for influenza patterns. Elveback et al. (1975, 1976a,b) introduced a variable infectiousness parameter (i.e. 4 % of clinical cases being highly infectious, 4 % of subclinical cases being moderately infectious, etc.). They found that these assumptions made no appreciable difference to the overall epidemic size or to the age-specific attack rates.

Though impressive and with great intuitive appeal, this modelling approach is not without its own problems. One is its very detailed structure. This suggests high specificity to the results, with unknown sacrifice in loss of generality. More important, however, is the problem of cost. Because of the prodigious number of calculations required, this model makes considerable demands on even a large computer. Elveback et al. (1976a) used a CDC 3300 system for their influenza studies, and quote a 1975 cost of $1.20 per epidemic (average computer processing time: approximately 1 minute). However, the stochastic nature of the model requires that a large number (at least 100) epidemics be run in order to provide detailed frequency distributions of predictions on the basis of each parameter set. Improvements in computer technology have reduced the real cost of such work in recent years, but it still remains high.

Elveback et al. (1975) present an excellent discussion of the principles and problems of modelling, with particular reference to these influenza studies. With regard to the highly stochastic nature of their models, they suggest that "the value of random variables lies entirely in impressing the consumer that we are studying influenza as they know it, without undue over-simplification". They recognized the need to lower the cost of the model operation by removing stochastic features which had little or no impact on the results, and by introducing analytical arguments in place of simulation, wherever possible. An important step in this direction was taken by Longini et al. (1978), working with Model VII as applied to influenza. They have in effect translated the model "back" into deterministic form, using expected values for parameters rather than Monte Carlo simulation of probability distributions, and shown that the deterministic results approximate very closely to the mean values derived through repeated stochastic simulations. The application of this deterministic model to studies of control strategies is discussed in Section 2.5.2.

2.4 Models of influenza in large populations

Many–perhaps most–epidemiological investigations of influenza have been based upon morbidity or mortality data from large populations. Such data are notoriously imprecise, with wide margins for errors and biases depending upon the notification or death certification system involved. Nonetheless, the impact of influenza in large populations is such as to be observable above a considerable amount of background "noise". And ever since the days of William Farr (e.g. 1847) epidemiologists have become increasingly clever at deciphering patterns of underlying phenomena from apparently very crude population data.

Chains of transmission are invisible in mass population data. Detailed social and geographic structure of a population is also generally lost, except for crude measures of occupation (sometimes available through death certificate data) and area. Thus models generally aim at descriptions or predictions of broad trends. Deterministic formulations are generally used, as the large populations are assumed to submerge the details of chance contacts between individuals (just as the prediction of 50 % heads becomes increasingly sound with repeated tossings of a coin). Furthermore, the large population sizes involved may make the Reed-Frost and mass action models equivalent (see Appendix D); and thus the mass action formulation has generally been chosen, on grounds of its greater mathematical simplicity. For all these reasons, we find that the dynamic models aiming at large populations are generally deterministic, mass-action formulations, with underlying assumptions of random-mixing homogeneous populations.

In addition to the dynamic models, there has been considerable interest in the application of descriptive, statistical models to influenza morbidity and mortality data.

2.4.1 General patterns of influenza epidemics in large populations

Influenza viruses may be persistently present within large populations; but it is the pattern of the periodic epidemics which has attracted most attention. These usually occur in winter, often beginning in December in the northern hemisphere. This timing presents a problem, as influenza occurs during the season when morbidity and mortality figures rise for many reasons: common colds, measles, mumps, chickenpox, etc. also rise during the colder months, and all-cause deaths rise during winters even when influenza is not observed. Several workers have argued that influenza morbidity and mortality increase after brief low-temperature periods, though the objective evidence for this is not overwhelming (Davey and Reid, 1972; McFarlane, 1976). Nonetheless, the careful student of influenza is acutely aware of the problems inherent in these seasonal phenomena which may hide or confound the impact of influenza.

Influenza epidemics, as manifested in either morbidity or mortality statistics, present as a rise and subsequent fall in incidence. It is a fact of observation that these epidemics, in common with most propagated epidemic phenomena, are often—though with interesting exceptions—quite symmetric in overall shape. Indeed, this observation led several early investigators to postulate that a fundamental "law" underlying propagative epidemics was such as to produce a bell-shaped "normal" curve. Subsequent workers came to recognize a consistent departure from such symmetry, however, and a general tendency for propagative epidemics to be "right-skew", i.e. for the initial rise in incidence to be more rapid than the subsequent fall. Fine (1979) discusses the histiory of this problem and of the important role played by mathematical models in its argument. The issues of the "shape" of epidemic curves, and of the reasons for these shapes, are still discussed today.

Spicer (1979) has recently drawn attention to these questions once again, with reference to influenza epidemics, in a study applying mass-action models to influenza mortality data in England and Wales. Spicer's investigation was stimulated by, and based upon, recent Russian work (discussed below, Section 2.4.2) modelling the spread of influenza across the USSR. It is an important paper in bringing this Russian work to the attention of a general Western audience. The model used is the simple, deterministic, discrete time, mass-action expression, with an added assumption that cases remain infectious for several days. The basic equation is thus phrased:

$$C_{(t+1)} = bS_t \sum_{t=0}^{6} C_{(t-T)} W_T \qquad (6)$$

where W_T is the probability that an individual is still *infectious*, T days after having become *infected*. (Compare this with equation 1, Section 2.1.1). Spicer apparently used a distribution of W_T suggested by Baroyan et al. (1977):

T =	days after infection:	0	1	2	3	4	5	6	7+
W_T =	proportion still infectious:	0	1.0	0.9	0.55	0.3	0.15	0.05	0.0

Spicer attempted to fit this model to weekly mortality data (weekly deaths as certified from influenza and influenzal pneumonia), as influenza morbidity is not routinely notified in the UK. This required an additional equation, defining the case fatality rates at specified intervals after onset of infection. Spicer set the overall case fatality rate at 2×10^{-4}, and proceeded to fit the model by least squares to mortality data on *unimodal* influenza epidemics in England and Wales, and in Greater London, during the period 1958-73.

Some of Spicer's results are shown in Figure 3. It will be noted that the fits are reasonably good, but that "generally speaking, the curve is too high at the beginning of the epidemic and too low at the end" (Spicer, 1979). Spicer suggests that it is the data rather than the model which is in error here, "since it is known that there is a tendency to under-notify at first and then over-notify in the later stages of the epidemic." Another explanation is possible: it is a property of the basic discrete time mass-action model that it gives a left-skew curve; thus it may be this feature of the model which explains Spicer's results. Fortmann and Florin (1975) and Fortmann (1976) have noted this peculiar property of the mass-action model; and it was precisely this unrealistic feature which led Brownlee to abandon mass-action theory back in 1906 (Fine, 1979). One might suppose that right-skew curves could be obtained by appropriate adjustment of the case duration function W_T; but Spicer found that the model's behavior appeared "not to be seriously affected by assumptions about the distribution of the infectious period."

Inspection of equation (6) reveals that the course of the predicted epidemic will be determined largely by the magnitude of b and S_0, i.e. the "transmission coefficient" and the initial number of susceptibles. This is so because the W_T function is assumed constant for all epidemics, and the initial number of cases, C_0, should be very small compared with S_0, the initial number of susceptibles. If this were so, then there is special interest in estimating the magnitude of b and S_0 early in an epidemic, as this should allow prediction of the subsequent epidemic course. Spicer thus estimated the product $b \cdot S$ for UK influenza epidemics, finding that it fell within the range of 3.9 to 7.7, the latter high value being associated with the H_3N_2 Hong Kong influenza of 1969-70.

It is worth noting that this product $b \cdot S_0$, called α by Spicer, is a re-phrasing of another recurrent theme in infectious disease theory, sometimes called the "case transmission ratio" or the "case reproduction rate". This is immediately apparent if we re-arrange Hamer's basic mass-action equation (1) as:

$$\frac{C_{t+1}}{C_t} = S_t \cdot b \tag{7}$$

FIGURE 3

Observed and estimated influenza mortality in England and Wales, by week, in selected years

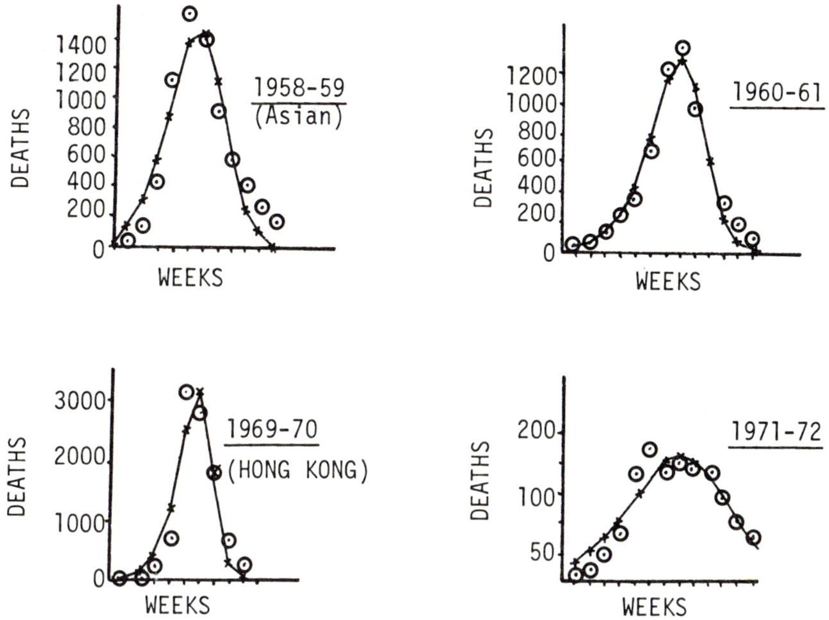

Observed data (— ⊙—) are from death certificates as reported to the Office of Population Censuses and Surveys. Estimated curves (— × —) represent best fit of adapted mass-action model to the observed data (Re-drawn from Spicer, 1979).

i.e. the product $S_t \cdot b$ is just the ratio of cases in successive time periods. If the time period is equal to the serial interval of the infection in question, then the product $S_t \cdot b$ is the average number of individuals infected by each case at time t. This parameter, the so-called "case transmission ratio", should fall during the course of an epidemic, as the number of susceptibles falls. It is maximum at the outset of an epidemic, i.e.

$$\frac{C_1}{C_0} = S_0 \cdot b = \alpha \qquad (8)$$

which is identical to what MacDonald (1957) called the "basic reproduction rate" in malaria, i.e. the average number of "successful" transmissions attributable to a single primary case introduced into a susceptible population.

We thus find ourselves dealing once again with basic mass-action theory. And the old concerns linger on: is it a valid or a reasonable model? Are fits such as those shown by Spicer (1979) or Fortmann (1976) "sufficiently" good? How does one judge? Firstly, looking at the shapes of the observed and predicted curves (e.g. Figure 3), one may suspect that William Farr's ancient, simple (and dynamically groundless) method of fitting symmetrical normal curves would provide even closer fits to the data than did the adapted mass-action model. And so would many other models. Secondly, is not the assumption of a constant *b* somewhat unreasonable, in its implication of homogeneity and random mixing for populations which obviously are not homogeneous and do not mix randomly? Thirdly, might not the consistent symmetry bias in the discrete mass-action reflect a fallacy of the model, and not of the data? Fourthly, given the evidence that social events such as school activities (Carey et al., 1958) and weather (e.g. McFarlane, 1976) may influence influenza epidemics, should we expect so simple a model as the mass-action to suffice? Finally, we may note that Spicer's application of the mass-action to influenza epidemic data has excluded "those whose curves showed obvious evidence of being bimodal". This reference is crucial, for real-life influenza epidemics are not infrequently undulating (Fortmann, 1976, recognizes this as a problem for mass-action theory), or in split waves (e.g. Chin et al., 1960), or bimodal (e.g. the H_2N_2 epidemic in the USA in 1957-58). It is essential to question the theoretical and practical basis of this mass-action concept, for its virtues of simplicity, elegance, or mathematical convenience are not in themselves assurance of biomedical validity.

2.4.2 Geographic spread

The ability of influenza viruses to move rapidly over vast areas of the earth's surface is well recognized. Maps illustrating the spread of pandemic H_2N_2 or H_3N_2 viruses around the world are found in many publications (e.g. Beveridge, 1977). No other pathogen manifests a capacity to travel so far, so fast. This property is both fascinating in terms of its underlying mechanism and important in terms of our ability to predict and to control the spread of these viruses.

Insofar as humans harbor and transmit influenza viruses, one might suppose that these viruses should travel where and when people travel. They should "go with the people". But this simple relationship has not been easy to demonstrate. N. T. J. Bailey tells the author (personal communication, 1980) that he has compared the apparent spread of pandemic viruses against statistics for population movement, but found no obvious relationship. Isaacs and Andrewes (1951), in discussing the pattern of influenza in 1950-51, noted "a surprising feature is that spread seemed to be directly geographical, rather than along main lines of communication." The apparent tendency for influenza to follow the compass is most evident in the annual transfer of influenza activity between northern and southern hemispheres, keeping up with the winter. Indeed, this property led Burnet to propose that influenza viruses depend upon "transequatorial swing" for their persistence in nature (cf. Andrewes, 1951). Improved surveillance has indicated that this is probably not so, at least in terms of virus persistence, but the problem of influenza's geography remains incompletely resolved.

One group of researchers has concentrated considerable attention on applications of mathematical models to this issue of influenza's spread. Their work has focussed upon the temporal pattern of influenza among large cities of the USSR, and has appeared in a series of publications since 1967 by Baroyan et al. and Rvachev et al. (see references). It is based on an assumption that the geographic spread of influenza is determined largely by population movements. The model is again of the mass-action type, though adapted so as to describe transmission between, as well as within, population centers.The model's predictions have been compared against morbidity data drawn from routine sickness absence records in the USSR.

I have found it difficult to assess this Russian work, because only a few of the publications are available in English translation. The modelling methods used, and the selection and nature of the observed data, are not always clear from the available material.

The basic framework consists of 128 sets of continuous-time mass-action equations, each set describing the rate of change in numbers of susceptibles and cases in a particular large population center (in general a city of over 100,000). Each set is very similar to the traditional Kermack-McKendrick equations (see Appendix B), with two additions. First, a special term is introduced to describe a frequency distribution of infectiousness extending just 6 days, in contrast to the Kermack-McKendrick assumption of constant recovery rate per unit time. This term has been explored by Spicer (1979), as expressed in equation (6) and discussed in Section 2.4.1. Second, the rates of change in numbers of susceptibles and of cases are increased by immigrants and decreased by emigrants between each of the several population centers, for each time period. The basic equations which most often appear in published discussions of this work are given and described in Appendix F. The resulting model is thus an inter-locking system of deterministic, mass-action equations purporting to describe influenza trends within and between 100 cities and 28 non-urban regions. Certain features of the model, especially relevant to its description of geographic trends, deserve further mention.

There has apparently been some exploration of applying different transmission factors, β ($=\lambda$ in the original authors' notation), to different cities. Baroyan et al. (1970) suggested that the β may be considered a product of two factors: β_1 describing the social structure of the population (which should vary between cities in the same epidemic but be constant within the same city for different epidemics); and β_2 describing the contagiousness of the agent (which should be constant for different cities during any single epidemic, but should vary between different epidemics). Though this is discussed, it appears that most simulations have assumed that β is constant for all cities.

The most interesting and important feature of the model is its method for describing the transfer of infection between populations. This is assumed to reflect the movement of people between the cities. Early versions of the model (pre-1970) described this by empirical equations implying that the daily immigration rate from city i to city j is equal to the product of the populations of the two cities times a factor estimated at 2^{-32}. We may note that this is, once again, basic mass-action theory, i.e. a rate of interaction between two populations being considered directly proportional to the product of the two populations concerned. In practical terms, it implies that, if both cities have populations of 100,000, then approximately 2.3 persons travel from i to j, and an equal number from j to i, per day. This may appear a rather low estimate. Just what such a migration parameter means is unclear, as there are major definitional problems in determining precisely what traffic flow may be relevant to influenza: for example, one might hypothesize that the risk of virus transfer from city i to city j was a function of the number of man-hours spent, per day, in city j by individuals who have been in city i within the past 6 days. In addition, one might suppose that the distance between population centers should enter into this equation, especially as the distances between the cities included in the analysis range from less than 100 to more than 3,000 kilometers. Despite this interpretive problem, Rvachev (1968) justified the early mass-action migration hypothesis by claiming that the predicted numbers of inter-city migrants correlated well with figures available through the Ministries of Transport and Civil Aviation. It is unclear whether that analysis was published.

More recent versions of the Rvachev-Baroyan model have superseded the original mass-action formulation for migration, and introduced a 128×128 matrix containing estimates of actual daily migration rates between cities. Numerical estimates were based upon official statistics for bus, rail, and air transport between population centers included in the model. Some of the practical problems which arose in adapting such statistics to the model's use are discussed in Baroyan et al.

(1977). Many cells of the matrix are effectively zero (i.e. the daily migration rate between some of the cities is considered negligible).

The model thus requires input data on the following parameters: the total population size of each city and the proportions susceptible, infected, and immune; the daily migration rates between each city in the network; the transmission factors β; and assumptions as to the frequency distribution of infection (infectiousness) duration. Since 1971, it has apparently been assumed that both the initial proportion susceptible, and the transmission factor β, are single constants for the entire country (Baroyan and Rvachev, 1977). Given this information, the computerized model provides a prediction of the subsequent incidence and prevalence through the course of the epidemic in the entire network of cities.

Early work with the model was discussed in relation to data on an epidemic which began in Leningrad in January 1965 and then spread to other cities in the USSR (Rvachev, 1968). At first, the only data available related to Leningrad in the early part of January, and to Moscow through the full course of the epidemic. It was found that the timing, magnitude, and shape of the Moscow epidemic course could be closely predicted on the basis of the initial Leningrad data. In 1970, data on other cities involved in the 1965 epidemic became available. Comparison of data from 19 additional cities, with predictions made in Rvachev's 1967 thesis, indicated good qualitative agreement (Baroyan et al., 1970). Some of these data are illustrated in Figure 4.

The nature of the data deserves comment. Observed statistics refer to what are called "DORM" ("Daily Officially Registered Morbidity"), apparently daily sickness absence claims (Baroyan et al., 1971). The specificity of the diagnoses is unclear from the publications available, but it appears that total sickness absences were used, rather than absences certified as due to influenza. With regard to this point, Baroyan et al. (1970) state: "We are not interested in the etiology of the outbreak... all these facts provide evidence that a new infecting factor 'x' has appeared, which could conditionally be called influenza." Though this may raise doubts as to the meaning of the observed data, their overall pattern is such as to indicate influenza as a major contributor. On the other hand, one should be cautious of possible confounding factors in such a situation. The observed data were affected by their origin as daily sickness absences. This leads to striking weekly cycles, with large excesses on Mondays, gradual decreases during the weekdays, and very low numbers at weekends. Special algorithms were thus written in order to modify the computer-predicted daily prevalence according to this weekday bias factor (Figure 5).

The published results of this work are impressive, and deserve

FIGURE 4

Observed (•••) and computer-predicted (———) morbidity in selected cities in the USSR, January-March, 1965. Only the early Leningrad data were used in setting the model.

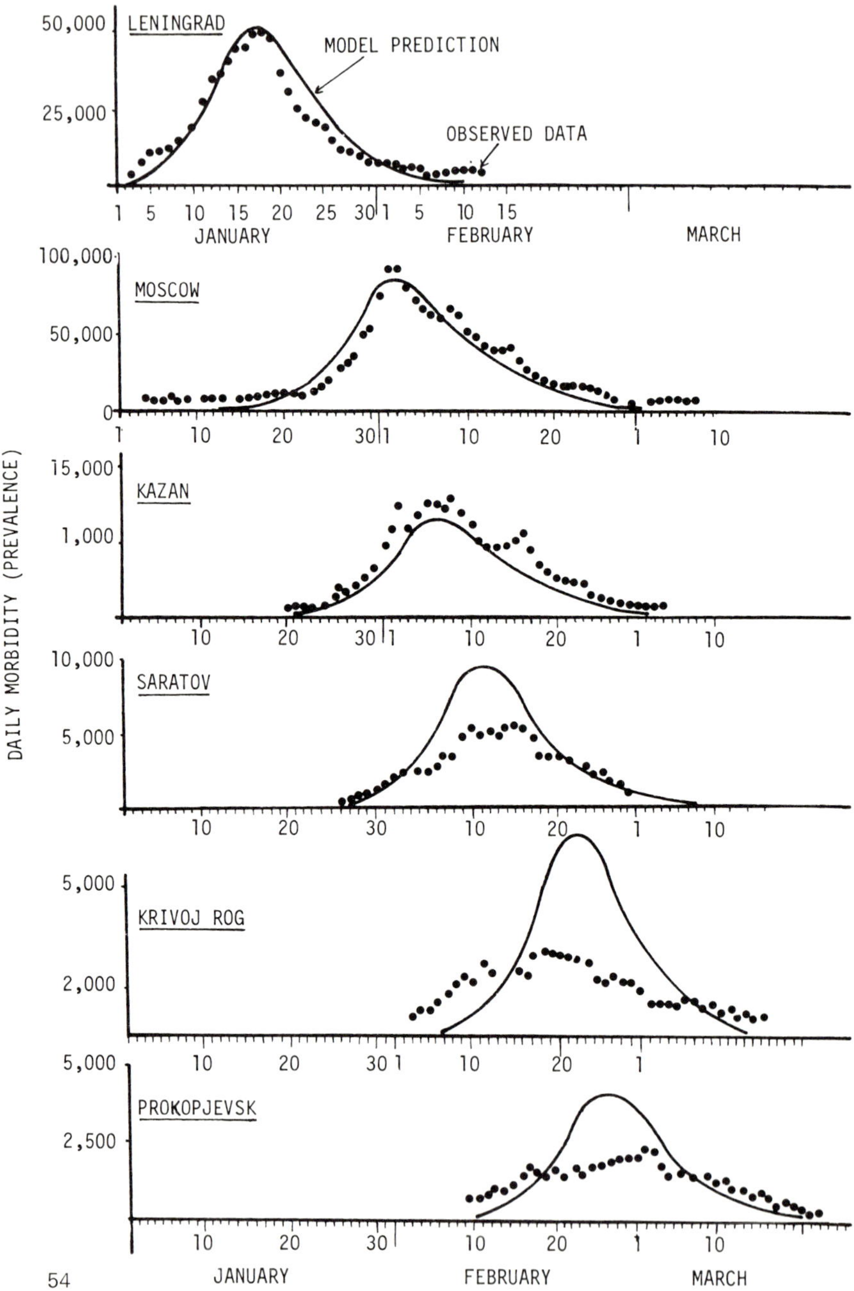

Redrawn from Baroyan et al., 1970.

FIGURE 5

Diagram showing adjustment of predicted "true" morbidity according to the Baroyan-Rvachev model, so as to take account of the weekly cycle in sickness absence reporting

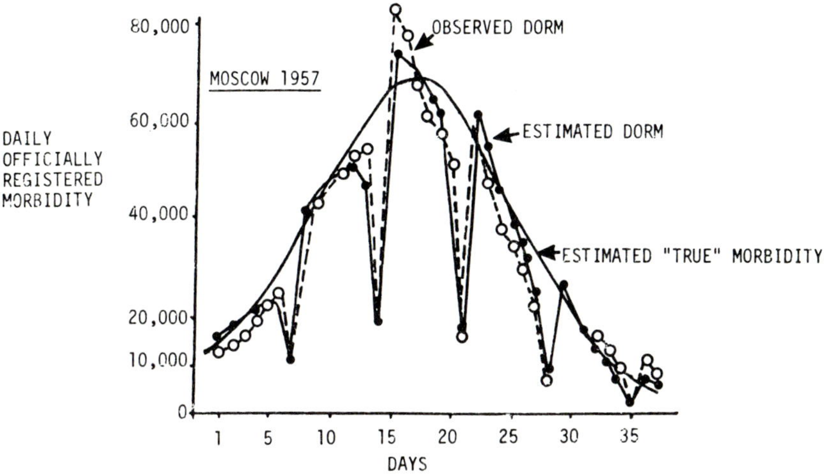

The jagged solid line represents this prediction adjusted for weekday-weekend biases. The dotted line represents actual reported Daily Officially Registered Morbidity (Redrawn from Baroyan et al., 1971).

epidemics for Krivoj Rog and for Prokopjevsk, both of which were apparently predicted—and observed—to peak approximately two weeks after the epidemics in the other cities. It should be noted that Krivoj Rog is in south-western USSR, not far from the early epidemics in Kiev, Donetsk, Gorlovka, and Zaporozje; whereas Prokopjevsk is some 3,000 kilometers to the east—yet itself only 200 kilometers from an early epidemic in Novosibirsk. The accuracy of the temporal prediction for these two cities would, if repeated and generalized, argue for the use of population movement statistics in descriptions and predictions of the spread of influenza. The fact that the two cities are so distant from one another, yet close to several other population centers with earlier epidemics, could provide evidence in the yet-unsettled argument as to whether—or to what extent—epidemic influenza follows people, the compass, the weather, or some other factor. On the other hand, it is unclear from the published material just how the 21 cities on which data were published were selected from the 128 cities included in the original model. And the critical reader may well be amazed that what is essentially a simple deterministic formulation would serve so well, against a background of so many anecdotes of the vagaries of influenza's behavior. The Rvachev-Baroyan model is interesting; its basis upon population movement statistics is a promising advance; and its attempt to model real data is laudable. But considerable critical examination of the work is required.

2.4.3 Excess mortality

The impact of influenza on a population is sometimes large. But how large? In what segment of population is it concentrated? How is it manifested? These questions are obviously of importance for determining the priority of influenza control (and research in general), as well as for directing control activities within a population. They have long been subjects of mathematical analysis. The models involved have generally been descriptive and statistical, rather than dynamic.

The great insight was William Farr's. Immediately upon becoming the first "Compiler of Abstracts" at the Office of the Registrar General of England and Wales, in 1837, Farr became aware of the regularity and predictability of mortality statistics. Therefore, when a severe influenza epidemic occurred in 1847, Farr was in a position to recognize a simultaneous marked increase in deaths attributed to bronchitis, pneumonia, asthma, and even some non-respiratory diseases. He deduced that these extra deaths either reflected misdiagnoses on the part of those who filled in the death certificates, or else represented "true" indirect effects of influenza. He went further. He compared the numbers of deaths recorded during influenza epidemics with the numbers of deaths if average mortality prevailed during the epidemic, and then estimated the number of influenza-attributable deaths by subtraction (Farr, 1847). This is the origin of the concept of "excess mortality", the recognition that the impact of an epidemic can be measured in terms of the excess of observed mortality, or morbidity, over the value expected for the period under consideration (Langmuir, 1976).[a]

Interest in this means of measuring the impact of influenza was revived after the great pandemic of 1918, largely by Selwyn Collins in the USA. Collins analyzed weekly all-cause and influenza-pneumonia mortality data from approximately 100 US cities, comparing these with expected values calculated as the median weekly numbers of deaths during previous non-epidemic years. Using this approach, Collins traced the course of epidemic influenza across the USA, and estimated that at least 250,000 excess deaths occurred during six minor influenza

[a] One might trace the excess mortality idea back to the Bills of Mortality in the 17th century, when the number of plague deaths was used as an indicator of epidemic plague. But this lacked the subtlety of Farr's insight.

epidemics between 1920 and 1929 (Collins, 1930). Like Farr, Collins (1932) also noted that "for every period in which there is a definite peak of excess mortality from influenza and pneumonia, there is a corresponding peak of excess mortality credited to causes other than influenza and pneumonia."

These methods were further developed by Serfling, again in the context of routine all-cause and pneumonia-influenza ("P & I") death reporting from cities in the USA (Eickhoff et al., 1961; Serfling, 1963). Like Farr and Collins, Serfling derived an expected value for P & I or all-cause mortality on the basis of data from previous non-epidemic years. But he discarded Farr's mean, and Collins' "moving median", in favor of a regression model fit by least squares to the weekly mortality data for the past five years, but omitting weeks with epidemic influenza (Appendix G). The regression equation includes sin and cosin terms, giving the line an appropriate annual periodicity. For almost 20 years, the CDC in Atlanta have used Serfling's equation to produce a baseline prediction for weekly P & I deaths, over the next 12 months, for approximately 120 US cities. The familiar graphs are usually published in October of each year in the Morbidity and Mortality Weekly Report (see Figure 6A). A dotted line is generally drawn 1.64 standard deviations above the regression curve. This is taken to be an "epidemic threshold". In theory, observed mortality in the absence of influenza should fall above this line, by chance, approximately once every 20 weeks, while "experience with this index has shown that an elevation above the epidemic threshold for 2 or more weeks usually indicates a rise in mortality of epidemiological interest" (Serfling, 1963). Tautologies notwithstanding, this measure has proven useful to the United States Public Health Service in recognizing influenza activity. It has also been used to estimate the total mortality cost of influenza epidemics, excess all-cause deaths during epidemic periods being calculated as the difference between the observed numbers and those expected on the basis of Serfling's model fitted to weekly all-cause mortality data during non-epidemic periods of the previous five years.

The Serfling model has been applied with minor variations to rather crude mortality data from several countries (Assaad et al., 1973; Peretjagina et al., 1977). More interesting have been several applications of the Serfling model to age- and cause-specific mortality data within the USA. Using this method it was noted that, although absolute excess P & I mortality generally has a U-shaped age distribution, being low between the ages of 5 and 40 and increasing greatly in older age groups, the percent excess due to H_2N_2 "Asian" influenza was quite constant for all age groups, except for a sharp peak among those aged 15-19 years during the first wave of the epidemic in late 1957 (Serfling et al., 1967). Houseworth and Spoon (1971) used a similar approach to reveal a

FIGURE 6

Weekly deaths attributed to pneumonia and influenza, in 121 cities of the USA

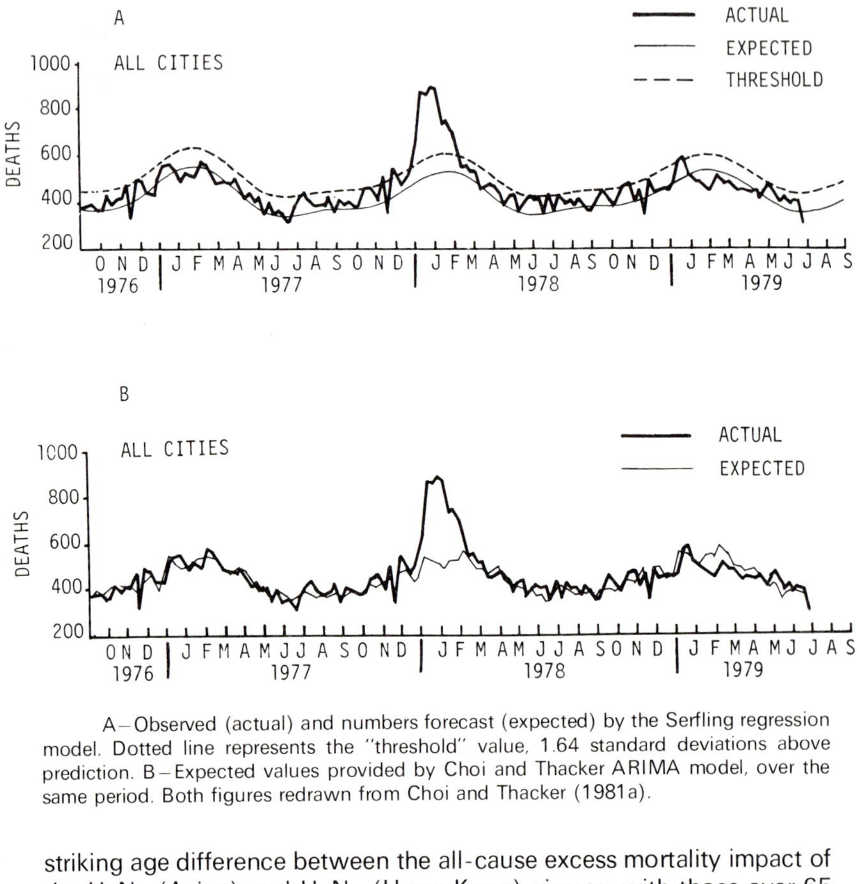

A – Observed (actual) and numbers forecast (expected) by the Serfling regression model. Dotted line represents the "threshold" value, 1.64 standard deviations above prediction. B – Expected values provided by Choi and Thacker ARIMA model, over the same period. Both figures redrawn from Choi and Thacker (1981a).

striking age difference between the all-cause excess mortality impact of the H_2N_2 (Asian) and H_3N_2 (Hong Kong) viruses, with those over 65 years of age suffering relatively more from the Asian than from the later Hong Kong virus, and an opposite trend among persons younger than 65 years. Houseworth and Langmuir (1974) found that more than half the influenza-associated excess all-cause deaths between 1957 and 1966 were attributable to diseases of the cardiovascular or nervous systems, and that the proportion attributable to respiratory causes ranged from 22% during mild outbreaks of influenza B to 38% in severe type A (H_2N_2) epidemics.

Despite such interesting applications, the Serfling model is not without problems. Because it is fitted to data on "non-epidemic" weeks only, it may tend to be biased too low. It assumes independence of all observations, thereby overlooking a logical association between adjacent points (i.e. the incidence of influenza in one week is to some extent dependent on the incidence in the previous week). It neglects the implications of altered reporting intervals at holiday periods. Its periodicity, although realistic, is guided more by trigonometry than by underlying biological processes. And its specificity for influenza activity is not perfect; at least once, the Serfling epidemic threshold has been crossed as a result of a heat wave in July (though the fault may be in the attribution of cause of death on death certificates, rather than in the model *per se*). These deficiencies have been discussed by Choi and Thacker (1981a,b), who have suggested an alternative to the Serfling model, based on Box-Jenkins-type time series analysis. The method goes under the rather forbidding name of the ARIMA ("auto-regressive integrated moving average") model (Figure 6B). This method does not assume independence of successive mortality data, but gives particular weight to points immediately preceding, and one year preceding, each prediction point. This introduces a pseudo-dynamic quality to the model (dependence of successive incidences). Choi and Thacker also show that proportional mortality (i.e. the *proportion* of all deaths due to pneumonia and influenza) provides a much more stable statistic, especially at holiday periods, than do the absolute numbers.

Two further conceptual problems arise in reference to the use of models for excess mortality studies. First is the use of the word "prediction". This term is often used to describe the baseline mortality trend extrapolated from previous non-epidemic year data, as in the operational use of the Serfling model. But this extrapolation is more a description of past mortality trends than a prediction of new ones. And it never, by its very nature, "predicts" epidemic influenza—it always "predicts" no epidemic! In this sense, it is a statement of the null-hypothesis. Secondly, the nature of the Serfling "epidemic threshold" should be noted. The phrase is used here not in the classical sense, as a threshold number of susceptibles which will lead to an epidemic increase in incidence (Appendix A), but for a level of mortality which is considered abnormally high and hence indicative of an epidemic. Despite its apparent objectivity, this criterion is arbitrary to the extent that it is based on a regression fit to mortality data which were originally *assumed* to be "non-epidemic". This arbitrariness is evident in Serfling's (1963) phrase, cited above, to the effect that the epidemic threshold identifies "mortality of epidemiologic interest". But different people find different things interesting. Sabin (1977) has suggested that too much emphasis has been placed upon the now conventional methods of excess mortality measured against non-epidemic baselines (but see Gregg et al., 1978; Kilbourne, 1978). Though his argument has missed the subtlety of Farr's insight of attributable excess during an influenza period, and overlooks Serfling's recognition that background trends must be incorporated in estimates of baseline mortality, Sabin's challenge has probably been salutory in encouraging reconsideration of the assumptions underlying—and the operational uses of—influenza baseline and excess mortality analyses. These discussions have recently led the CDC to favor Choi and Thacker's ARIMA approach, rather than that of Serfling, for their routine influenza analyses.

Though simple baseline mortality estimates will continue to be useful in operational planning, and in measurement of epidemic size, detailed questions of influenza's impact on human populations may better be answered through alternative statistical approaches which introduce additional variables known to be associated with influenza (e.g. Alling et al., 1981; Clifford et al., 1977; Tillett et al., 1980).

2.5 Operational models

Norman Bailey ends the second edition of his book on mathematical epidemiology (1975) by paraphrasing Marx—saying that it is all very well for philosopher-mathematicians to describe the world in various ways, but that the real problem is to change it (might we add: favorably). The bottom line of research should be action. The discussion above has concentrated largely upon models in a research context, for describing influenza or for investigating its underlying mechanisms. What about the more practical operational uses of models in public health, specifically in the prediction of influenza activity and in the guidance of its control?

2.5.1 Models for prediction of influenza

Prediction is a favorite pastime of gamblers, mystics, and influenza specialists. The dramatic nature of influenza epidemics and their tantalizing, almost regular recurrences encourage this.

The use of mathematics in this art of epidemic forecasting dates back to William Farr's signal success in predicting the course of a rinderpest epidemic on the strength of a simple algorithm based on initial incidence data (Brownlee, 1915; Farr, 1866; Fine, 1979). Indeed it is no coincidence that it was Farr's worshipful follower, John Brownlee, who would write a paper entitled "The next epidemic of influenza", basing his prediction upon periodic analysis of influenza mortality data (Brownlee, 1919). The predicted epidemic did not occur (Brownlee, 1923).

Brownlee's was an attempt at long-range forecasting–the prediction of an influenza epidemic's occurrence before the fact. Others have tried. These attempts were reviewed by the Commission on Acute Respiratory Diseases (1946), who themselves suggested that the mechanism underlying influenza's cycle was analogous to that in measles, a "balance of immunes and susceptibles". Their prediction, based on an implicit mathematical analysis, also failed. Subsequent virological work has revealed the antigenic shift mechanism underlying pandemic influenza, and handed over the challenge of long-range prediction to the molecular biologists. Several have not hesitated to suggest that shifts could be predicted on the basis of virus genome mutation rates, and upon selection pressures imparted by "herd immunity" (e.g. Fazekas de St Groth, 1975; Masurel, 1976). And Hope Simpson (1978) has suggested that the sunspot cycle may provide an indicator of the critical shift mutations. Gamblers, mystics, and influenza specialists... .

If prediction of epidemics before the fact still seems elusive, there may be a greater chance of success in predicting the subsequent course of an epidemic, once it has begun. If it should prove that influenza epidemics follow a predictable temporal or spatial course–for example, the sort of curve defined by a mass-action equation–then one might have some confidence in predicting the trend of an epidemic.

The fitting–even close fitting–of one or another model to a completed set of epidemic incidence data is not sufficient to demonstrate predictability in the "true" or operationally useful sense. What is required is that a model be fitted only to data collected in the early part of an epidemic. The extrapolation or prediction on the basis of this initial fitting should then be compared with the actual observed remainder of the epidemic. This is the method used by William Farr in 1866, in what is perhaps the only example of successful epidemic prediction in history–as Farr had the courage to publish his forecast before the event. Indeed open, prior publication is the only convincing demonstration of predictive capability.[a]

The only workers to have concentrated on forecasting the subsequent course of an already initiated influenza epidemic are Rvachev, Baroyan, et al., who claim success in predicting the temporal and spatial spread of certain influenza epidemics across the USSR, on the basis of the early course and location (city) of an initial outbreak. The

[a] It should be noted that the predictive power of Farr's models (which were based upon simple assumptions of constant second or third ratios between consecutive incidences) was examined by Evans (1876). This investigation revealed wide variation in predicted courses, dependent upon the assumptions and the extent of initial data available.

model used in these studies, and the story of its application to data collected in several cities of the USSR in 1965, were described in Section 2.4.2. Since the original studies on the 1965 epidemic, the model has been applied to morbidity data for several different years (Baroyan and Rvachev, 1977). Data from cities first hit by an epidemic are used to derive estimates of the within-city mass-action transmission coefficient, β, and the proportion initially susceptible in the population, i.e. x_0/P. A least-squares type of procedure is used for this, but the rules for the calculation, and for the selection of an optimal pair of an infinite array of β and x_0/P values, are not clear to me. The values are then assumed constant for all cities included within the model. Equations similar to those in Appendix F are then used to provide deterministic predictions of the time of appearance and course of consequent epidemics in each city of the "transport network". The accuracy of the predictions for the several cities has been measured in terms of the errors in predicting the day of peak morbidity (ΔT = difference in days between predicted and observed peak) and errors in predicting the extent of peak daily morbidity (ΔH = ratio of predicted to actual peak daily morbidity).

Baroyan and Rvachev (1977) discuss the application of the model to the Hong Kong influenza epidemic which swept the USSR between December 1968 and March 1969. Though the epidemic apparently appeared initially in Dushanbe and Frunze, the first city for which sufficient data were available was Kuibyshev, where recorded morbidity rose above baseline on 20 January 1969 (this is called the "prognostic point", but just how it is determined is not clear). The model was then fitted to data from Kuibyshev (the fitting procedure is not fully described), giving estimates of $\beta = 2.14$ and $x_0/P = 0.25$ (thus implying that 25% of the population was susceptible to morbidity-producing infection at the start of the epidemic). On the basis of these parameter values, and the model's assumptions of within- and between-city "contact", the rest of the epidemic was predicted. This apparently included a backwards projection to describe the earlier epidemic in Frunze, which peaked on 25 December 1968. Baroyan and Rvachev (1967) present the results of the model's predictions for 39 cities diagrammatically, as in Figures 7 and 8. With regard to the ΔT, ΔH plot in the upper half of Figure 7, the authors considered the temporal prediction good in 38 of the 39 cities, and the overall predictions good in 24. The lower half of Figure 7 shows the accuracy of predictions made by an alternative method, called "formal extrapolation", though just what this means is not clear. It is interesting that this method appeared consistently to predict peaks 15 days too early.

Figure 8 presents the overall observed and model-predicted morbidity pattern attributed to Hong Kong influenza in 40 cities, adjusted for the weekday bias of sickness absence reporting. Once again,

FIGURE 7

Diagram illustrating the accuracy of predictions of the spread of Hong Kong influenza across the USSR, according to the Rvachev-Baroyan model

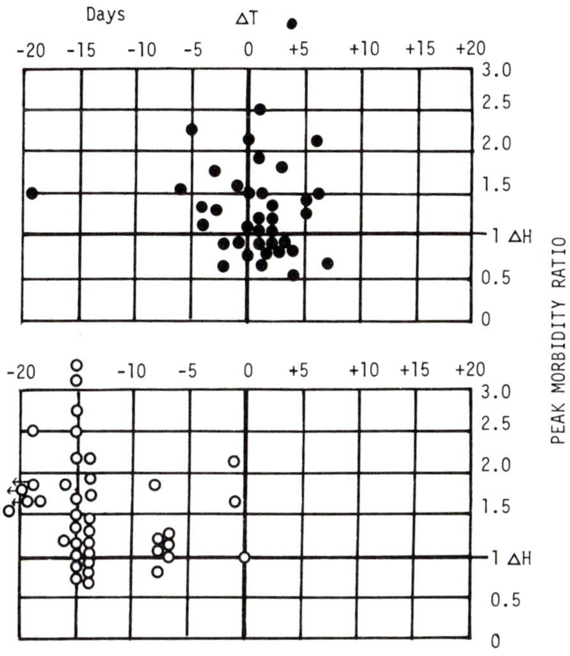

The ΔT scale gives the difference in days between the observed and expected epidemic peak, for each city. The ΔH scale gives the ratio of observed to predicted epidemic heights (maximum daily morbidity). The top graph represents model predictions and actual data for 1969. The bottom graph represents an alternative method of prediction, called "formal extrapolation", against actual data for 1969. (Redrawn from Figure 10 of Baroyan and Rvachev, 1977.)

the correspondence is striking. It is unfortunate that Baroyan and Rvachev's (1977) account does not include detailed discussion of the actual data and of the calculations involved in this work. Some of this important detail may be included in the monograph by Baroyan et al. (1977), which is not yet available in English.

Baroyan (personal communication, 1980) informs me that, since 1971, the Rvachev-Baroyan model has had "practical applications on the whole territory of the country. In particular,... the model really predicts the officially registered daily morbidity of influenza for the whole period of

FIGURE 8

Observed (dotted line) and computer-predicted (solid line) daily morbidity during Hong Kong influenza epidemic in 40 cities of the USSR

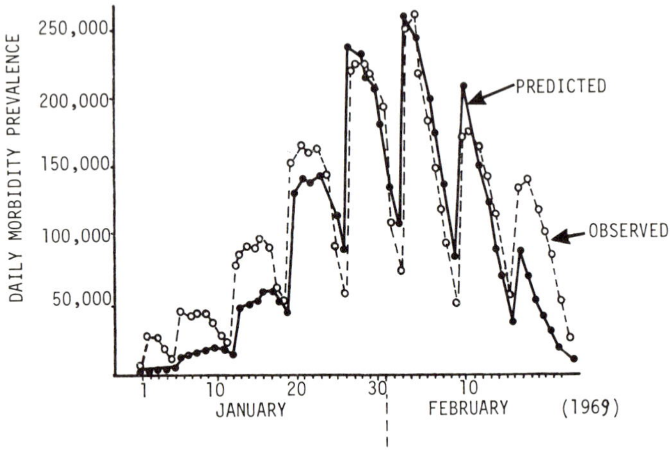

(Redrawn from Baroyan and Rvachev, 1977.)

the epidemic." Further clarification of such an achievement, and of its uses in public health planning, are awaited with considerable interest.

With reference to the practical implications of the geographic spread of influenza viruses, we should recognize that jet planes introduce a means for very rapid and very distant transfer of virus (e.g. Moser et al., 1979). Indeed, "jet spread" was a major worry of epidemiologists faced with the prospect of a swine 'flu epidemic in the USA in 1976 (Neustadt and Fineberg, 1978).

2.5.2 Models for control of influenza

An argument which is often voiced in support of work on models is that they should be useful in determining control strategies. In principle, models provide easily manipulated systems against which different control approaches can be tested and optimized. To what extent do the available mathematical models of influenza help us in this important sphere?

The control of a communicable disease such as influenza may be based on one or a combination of approaches: prophylactic immunization distributed so as to protect either individuals or communities; chemoprophylaxis with a drug, such as amantadine, to protect exposed individuals or communities; or measures to reduce contact and virus transmission within a community, such as isolation of cases, closure of schools or meetings, restriction of population movement, or even the wearing of face masks. The choice of methods is by no means straightforward. It must be debated, made, and carried out in the context of the many social, ethical, and economic constraints of the real world. More importantly, it rests upon even more fundamental questions concerning influenza control—someone must first decide whether to control it at all, how much can be invested, who is to be protected and for how long, etc.

Models may be useful in the preliminary phases of a control program. Because influenza epidemics are so short-lived, advance warning of their arrival is helpful if not absolutely necessary to their control. Thus there is a clear role for accurate predictive models as discussed in Section 2.5.1. Long-range prediction is essential if a vaccine is to be used against a new shift virus, as at least six months are required for preparation, testing, and production of a new vaccine. (The 1976 swine influenza episode in the USA is a now classic example of this situation—see Neustadt and Fineberg, 1976.) Shorter-range predictions are useful for control of minor drift viruses, providing time to order supplies and to prepare a program.

Given the imminence or just the annual possibility of an epidemic, the basic question arises: who is to be protected, and at what cost to the community? Is the goal to reduce absenteeism at school or in the work force (for which purpose many industries encourage routine vaccination), or is it to reduce excess mortality (for which purpose several countries offer routine influenza vaccination to elderly and "high-risk" individuals)? Or is it to minimize the work load on the health services? Certainly the work on excess mortality models is relevant to such questions.

These complicated but fundamental questions are generally overlooked in the literature on mathematical models for disease control strategies. Only Elveback, Fox, and their colleagues have addressed them with reference to influenza (*vide infra*). Most workers have confined themselves to a much simpler and less real problem: assuming there is a randomly mixing population and a contagious agent, how many (what proportion) should be immunized in order to prevent an epidemic increase in incidence? The most common solution of this problem traces back to the simple mass-action and epidemic threshold model of Hamer (Appendix A). The argument is as follows:

According to the mass-action equation (1), the ratio of incident cases in successive serial intervals is given as in equation (7), i.e.

$$\frac{C_{t+1}}{C_t} = S_t \cdot b \qquad (7)$$

In other words, the proportional increase in incidence between times t and $t+1$ is given by the product of the number of susceptibles at time t (S_t) times the transmission coefficient (b). This product has been called the "case transmission ratio" or the "case reproduction rate" by different authors. According to theory (virtually by definition) an epidemic begins to disappear, or does not occur, if this product is less than unity. Thus the goal of a mass immunization program should be to reduce the number of susceptibles at least until $S_t \cdot b < 1$. For example, given a case transmission ratio $S_t \cdot b = 4$ (i.e. a four-fold increase of incidence each serial interval), then immunization of 75% susceptibles would reduce the case transmission ratio to unity, implying constant incidence; and immunization of more than 75% should bring an immediate fall in incidence, i.e. $C_{t+1}/C_t < 1$.

Precisely this argument has been presented by many authors, and has been suggested for influenza control in at least three recent publications (Damms et al., 1976; Fortmann, 1976; Smith, 1976). It is intimately tied to the concept of "herd immunity", which is widely referred to in the literature on immunization strategies. According to the most common convention, a population or "herd" is "immune" when a sufficient proportion of its susceptibles has been protected, so that $S_t \cdot b < 1$, i.e. incidence falls.

This simple concept of "herd immunity", based on the mass-action model, is elegant and appealing; but it can be seriously misleading. Its failings are basically those of the mass-action model itself—real populations are *not* made up of identical homogeneous individuals, and do *not* mix at random. Just how far these assumptions lie from the reality of influenza transmission has been stressed repeatedly in this review. The literature contains many instances in which infections have been maintained despite the fact that the proportion immunized in the overall community was higher than that predicted to give "herd immunity", evidently because the agent was being transmitted selectively within an unprotected subset of the population (e.g. Smith, 1976).[a] Another problem with the simplistic interpretation of herd immunity is its emphasis on proportions rather than absolute numbers of susceptibles; e.g. if 100 susceptibles are required to maintain an agent over a period of time, these 100 may occur in an unvaccinated population of 100, or in a population of 1,000 which is 90% immune. Whether the latter population can maintain transmission will depend upon the mixing characteristics of the population. Fox et al. (1971) discuss these

[a] Perhaps the best examples of the failure of the simplistic herd immunity concept were revealed in the course of the WHO smallpox eradication program in Asia. High immunization levels were often concentrated in certain segments of populations, allowing unimpeded transmission in less thoroughly covered social groups (e.g. Henderson, 1972).

problems with the simple herd immunity concept, pointing out that "the question 'what proportion of the population should be immunized to prevent an epidemic?' is not answerable" without a considerable amount of information concerning the size, structure, and epidemiological characteristics of the population concerned.

Detailed decisions as to optimum immunization – or other control – policy therefore (and obviously) require detailed information as to the size, age structure, social structure, contact pattern, and immunological history of the population in question. The only workers who have attempted to construct models with such detailed information are Elveback, Fox, and their colleagues. Their approach, based on the simulation of daily events in a highly structured theoretical community, was described in Section 2.3.2. Such a method allows detailed exploration of virtually any manner of control, directed at any segment of the population at any point in the course of an epidemic. For example, the authors have investigated the implications of school closure on the pattern of epidemics simulated in their Model IV (Elveback et al., 1971). This is done by reducing the within-school contact rate to zero for the period of closure. Though their published discussion in this case related to Coxsackie virus epidemics, the modelling technique is applicable to influenza as well. Their 1975 and 1976 papers were devoted to applications of Model VII to influenza control studies, and concentrate largely on the implications of delivering different vaccines (killed or live, with different efficacies and immunity induction periods) at different times (before or after actual onset of an H_2N_2 or H_3N_2 epidemic) to different segments of the simulated population (school and pre-school groups in particular). The predictions compared favorably with limited available data on comparisons of different control strategies in similar populations (e.g. Monto et al., 1969).

The flexibility of the Elveback et al. approach is virtually limitless. Though they have not applied their model to investigate the effectiveness of amantadine, or wearing face masks, such interventions need only be specified in quantitative terms for their effects to be open to exploration. Anything which can be formulated can be simulated. On the other hand, several drawbacks of this detailed simulation approach were mentioned in Section 2.3.2 and should be reiterated here.

First is the question of the applicability of the results to communities which differ markedly in size and structure to that used in the published simulations. In principle this problem requires only further exploration of the model with different population assumptions. But this will be expensive.

Second is the problem of cost itself. The fully stochastic simulation approach of Elveback et al. requires between 100 and 200 dollars' worth of computer time to explore a single set of assumptions. Extensive exploration of different community structures and control strategies is thus prohibitively expensive. A major advance in this regard has been made by Longini et al. (1978), who have shown that the structured community model can be formulated in deterministic terms, and that the deterministic results are very close to the mean values obtained by the far more expensive stochastic simulation procedure. In addition, Longini et al. have introduced an optimization routine, which explores different allocations of vaccine in order to minimize some cost variable (either per capita expense or total mortality). Their results suggest that optimal allocation of vaccine resources will depend upon several variables, including the behavior of the wild virus (e.g. H_2N_2 versus H_3N_2), the amount of vaccine available, and the output "cost" variable which is to be optimized. This work represents an important methodological advance in the application of models to problems of disease control.

Finally, there is the problem of validating the model. This is a requirement for all models, but may be especially difficult for those of Elveback et al., because of the large amount of detail included in the model's structure. The enhanced specificity of the models also enhances the problems of validation.

3. Prospectus

Having surveyed the available literature on models as applied to influenza, thoughts inevitably turn to the logical directions for such work in the future. There follow several brief, personal—and inevitably prejudiced—opinions on this important question of "what next?".

1. *Family studies.* The potential usefulness of family studies of influenza has not been exhausted. Additional careful descriptive and secondary attack rate studies are most required; but the application of available models to such data would provide a helpful framework for consideration of several questions of fundamental importance to an understanding of the behavior of influenza viruses. For example, the time distribution of influenza cases within families, as published by several authors (Hope Simpson, 1979; Hope Simpson and Sutherland, 1954; Jordan et al., 1958), has not been satisfactorily explained. Another question is that of the low intra-family secondary attack rates which have been found by many authors, in contrast to very high secondary attack rates in other close contact situations (e.g. Chin et al., 1960; Davis et al., 1970; Jordan et al., 1958; Moser et al., 1979). To what extent subclinical infections, mis-classifications of primary and secondary cases, extra-familial transmission, or differential infectiousness ("superspreaders")

may be responsible for these anomalies has not been clarified. A recent paper by Kemper (1980), on sources of error in household secondary attack rate measures, is very relevant to this problem. In addition, there is the untapped potential of detailed family studies for comparing the epidemiological behavior of different influenza viruses.

The models discussed in Section 2.2 are appropriate for the investigation of such questions. What is needed is their critical application to carefully collected data. Ideally, the data collection should include serological tests in order to pick up subclinical case links in the chains of transmission. Certainly a clear distinction should be made between cases of infection and/or disease. Recent advances in sero-epidemiological techniques (e.g. Schild et al., 1977) should facilitate this. Data collection should aim at a finer time resolution than the nearest day. Just as the epidemiological analysis of food poisoning episodes is often dependent on hourly data, the precise study of influenza within families may require onset data to the nearest 12, if not six, hours. The study by Moser et al. (1979) shows that 12-hour precision is feasible and useful. Finally, the data should include as thorough a description as possible of the full epidemiological context of the family cases: i.e. data on the age, sex, "occupation", vaccination history, etc., of the individuals concerned; and data on the geographic and temporal position of family outbreaks within a community epidemic as a whole. Most importantly, the manipulation and interpretation of the models applied to such data should be critical, with a sense of studying influenza rather than of studying models or statistics.

2. *Small community studies.* Though the exploration of simple homogeneous community random-mixing models is highly useful in a teaching context, their appropriateness for description of actual small community data on influenza is questionable. Because human groups are in general non-homogeneous, and do not mix at random, departures of epidemic patterns from simple mass-action or Reed-Frost assumptions are to be expected. Thus the applications of such models would seem most appropriate and productive only if the detailed emphasis were placed on the *departures* rather than on the consistencies of models and data. This important principle of scientific-statistical logic, that it is by refuting ($p < 0.05$) rather than supporting ($p > 0.05$) an hypothesis that progress is made, is unfortunately absent from much of the literature on modelling.

The heterogeneous community non-random mixing models of Elveback et al. provide another approach to the study of influenza, which should be explored by other workers. The recent work by Longini et al. (1978) reduces the high computing cost of such modelling, and removes this barrier to their propagation. There is probably scope for further improvements in the methodology of such models so as to preserve the stochastic features of the general models at much-reduced monetary cost. Elveback has informed the author (personal communication, 1980) that a full monograph is planned discussing these models and their computing implications. Such a monograph would be an extremely valuable contribution to the epidemiology literature, and should be encouraged.

There is a need for considerable further exploration, using heterogeneous-community models, of the implications of different community sizes and structures for epidemiological patterns. Only by such investigation will any generality in such results become evident. It seems important to tie the exploration of Elveback-type models to detailed field studies of real communities, in order to validate input parameters (social structure assumptions and within-group contact rates) and output patterns (group-specific attack rates, overall epidemic trends). Elveback et al. (1976) state that their contact rates were selected partly on the basis of information in the literature, and partly on the basis of the implications for the model's output. But they are not unique sets. It would thus be of interest to explore the ranges of these parameters which are consistent with realistic epidemic prediction and with actual field data. Further discussion of these rates, and of reasons for their differences, would be helpful (e.g. why was the total community contact rate higher for H_3N_2 Hong Kong than for H_2N_2 virus? If this reflected differences in age-specific immunity, such differential susceptibility could be introduced directly into the model. If it reflected differences in virus behavior, it is of interest to know how). The fact that the Elveback-type model can examine such detailed epidemiological equations is eloquent testimony of its power.

3. *Large population studies*. Models of influenza in large communities should be more adventurous than their forbears. The published models purporting to describe large population trends have all been based on simple mass-action homogeneity and random mixing assumptions—the only exception being the inter-city migration factor introduced in the Rvachev-Baroyan models, but still in terms of the mass-action model. The obvious inconsistency between these assumptions and reality are argued away on grounds of mathematical expediency or because it is hoped that large numbers will overwhelm the heterogeneity and chance effects. It is not clear that this is so. The assumption should be challenged. It would seem worthwhile to explore heterogeneous population non-random mixing assumptions within these models, perhaps using an approach analogous to that of the Elveback et al. models.

Rather than continue to force influenza into simple epidemic theory, an effort should be made to tackle some of the major puzzles of influenza patterns in large communities—the bimodal or undulating incidence pattern which is often observed, the apparent disappearance of virus for several months from large areas, or the recent recognition of widespread co-circulation of different shift viruses. Simulation techniques which incorporate important influencing factors such as weather patterns, seasonal factors (e.g. school terms), or social and geographic structure may be useful here.

Most models have focussed upon the problem of epidemic influenza, overlooking the fascinating issue of its endemicity—the persistence of single or co-circulating virus types between epidemics. The apparent disappearance of influenza viruses from large populations, for periods of several months, and their sudden reappearance over wide areas, has led to hypotheses of latency (Hope Simpson, 1979) or even—the sublime and the ridiculous—of repeated virus introduction from space (Hoyle and Wickramasinghe, 1979). To what extent the pattern may be explicable on the basis of more simple assumptions of seasonal changes in contact rates (as in measles), coupled with a high proportion of subclinical cases, has not been sufficiently explored. The modelling approaches of Bartlett (e.g. 1960) and of Yorke et al. (e.g. 1979) would seem especially appropriate to these questions of influenza virus persistence.[a]

The role of geographic spread in determining influenza patterns is a critical area for further exploration. The introduction of population-movement statistics into models of this problem, in the Rvachev-Baroyan model, is a useful advance in this regard.[b] There is considerable intuitive appeal in this approach, and it would be very satisfying if the method were confirmed. The predictions of these models should be examined critically, in the context of alternative—or additional, or confounding—explanations for influenza spread associated with weather

[a] I suspect that the "solution" to this problem is intimately tied to measures of the transmissibility of influenza viruses, and to seasonal changes in this transmissibility as affected by social and weather factors. Given the very short latent period of influenza, the viruses could not persist except in very large populations if their transmission potential (as measured by secondary attack rates, for example) were as high as those for measles or smallpox. It is of interest to explore whether the maintenance strategy of the influenza virus is dependent upon (a) the vast size of the world's human population, (b) a low average, low variance infectiousness potential, (c) a low average but high variance infectiousness, and/or (d) repeated antigenic shifts or drifts.

[b] It is of interest to note a methodological analogy between the Rvachev-Baroyan and Elveback et al. approaches. Both treat the total population of interest as made up of different subgroups (cities or social groups, respectively) with potentials for virus transfer both within and between them.

patterns, chance effects, or "transequatorial swing". An English translation is currently being prepared of a lengthy document describing the methods of this Russian work (Baroyan et al., 1977). Its availability hopefully will encourage a more thorough and critical examination of the theoretical and technical approach used. There have been several recent advances in methodology for modelling geographic patterns of disease, and these might well be applied to influenza (e.g. Bailey, 1980; Cliff et al., 1981).

The concept of excess mortality models has remained the same since Farr's original work in 1847, the main difference being in whether a mean, median, Fourrier term, or auto-regression line provides the baseline. Though a major function of these models in recent years has been to provide a signal of influenza activity "of epidemiologic interest" (Serfling, 1963), their use in assessing the magnitude and manifestation of influenza's impact (e.g. Houseworth and Langmuir, 1974; Houseworth and Spoon, 1971) is probably more important. Further work to answer the recent criticisms of excess mortality measures (e.g. Sabin, 1977) would be useful. This should include adaptations of excess mortality assessments to non-epidemic periods, and development of highly sensitive and *specific* methods for monitoring influenza virus activity.

4. *Operational models*. The recent swine 'flu episode in the USA has highlighted the tremendous practical importance of accurately predicting epidemic influenza. I am skeptical that mathematical models can be of much use in the long-term prediction of pandemics (improved virological and epidemiological surveillance is most important in this regard); but geographic spread models may have some practical function in short-term prediction.

As far as models for determining control strategies are concerned, the recent work of Elveback et al. represents an impressive advance towards an operationally feasible methodology. Considerable further work should be done in exploring these simulation models and adapting them to different circumstances. The development of simplified versions of these models, which could be run on small computers such as are becoming increasingly and widely available, would be a very useful contribution. They might then be used both in teaching and in health department operations offices. The models should be adapted so as to simulate real communities in which field studies have or will be carried out, in order to assess the predictive accuracy of the models. Conversely, field studies could be organized in populations simulated by the model. I believe that such efforts would be the most productive investment towards making epidemiological modelling an operationally useful exercise. Even if the models do not end up being used for day-to-day decision making, their widespread appreciation would encourage a more rational and effective approach to influenza control than is practiced today, where goals are generally not clearly defined, and preventive measures are often not vigorously encouraged.

The influenza models discussed in this review provide a nice illustration of a fundamental paradox in modelling work—the tension between the simplicity of elegant abstraction on one hand and the complexity of messy reality on the other. A crucial issue is just how much complexity need be introduced into a model for it to prove "useful". The simple random-mixing mass-action theory has dominated theoretical epidemiology for many years—largely, perhaps, because these models were tractable and elegant, and because more realistic formulations were unmanageable by mathematical analysis. Modern computer technology has broken this stalemate, however, as machine simulation techniques allow exploration of highly complex formulations. This has made possible the interesting approaches of Rvachev-Baroyan and of Elveback et al. The latter are of special interest as the non-homogeneous community, non-random mixing models combine an intuitively satisfying realism with a readily understood modelling technology. It is clear that the "usefulness" criterion for models changes, in this evolution, from that of the elegant insight to something with greater practical and operational potential. This is an important step towards moving mathematical epidemiology back from its recent sojourn as a branch of mathematics, towards its "rightful" home as a branch of epidemiology.

4. Mathematical appendix

A. Mass-action models and the epidemic threshold

The simple mass-action model of Hamer is phrased:

$$C_{t+1} = C_t \cdot S_t \cdot b \tag{A1}$$

Clearly, the number of cases will increase ($C_{t+1} > C_t$) if $S_t \cdot b > 1$, i.e. $S_t > \frac{1}{b}$. This $1/b$ is thus a measure of the epidemic threshold number of susceptibles.

This simple model implies that each case lasts for only a single time period (serial interval). This may not be the situation in influenza, however, in which the serial interval may be shorter than the infectious period. The model is easily adapted to this:

$$C_{t+1} = C_t + C_t \cdot S_t \cdot b - C_t \cdot r \tag{A2}$$

where r = the proportion of infectious cases which recover in one time period (serial interval).
Rearranging terms, this gives:

$$\frac{C_{t+1}}{C_t} = 1 + S_t b - r \qquad \text{(A3)}$$

In order for the number of cases to increase, i.e. $(C_{t+1}/C_t) > 1$, we must have

$$S_t > \frac{r}{b} \qquad \text{(A4)}$$

This statement, that the epidemic threshold number of susceptibles is given by the ratio of the recovery rate to the transmission factor, is analogous to the famous "threshold theorem" of Kermack and McKendrick (1927).

B. The Kermack-McKendrick continuous time mass-action equations

Though Ross (e.g. 1915) was apparently the first to phrase the mass-action principle in continuous time form, the classical development of this approach occurred in the hands of Kermack and McKendrick (1927). Using x, y, and z for the numbers of susceptibles, infective cases, and recovered-removed cases, respectively, and β and γ for the transmission and recovery-removal rates, respectively, they set up the following equations:

$$dx/dt = -\beta xy \qquad \text{(A5)}$$

$$dy/dt = \beta xy - \gamma y \qquad \text{(A6)}$$

$$dz/dt = \gamma y \qquad \text{(A7)}$$

Note that this assumption of a constant recovery-removal rate implies that the duration of cases has a negative exponential distribution. As with the discrete time equations, the continuous model predicts an epidemic (i.e. an increase in incidence) when $dy/dt > 0$, i.e. when x, the number of susceptibles, exceeds γ/β.

C. Derivation of the basic Reed-Frost equation

The basic Reed-Frost model expression is derived as follows. As in the simple mass-action equation, time is divided into discrete units, each equal to the serial interval of the infection in question. Infected individuals are infectious only during the time period following their having contracted the infection. The population mixes at random. S_t, C_t, and C_{t+1}

represent numbers of susceptibles and of cases during time periods t and $t+1$, respectively. Then:

p = probability that a susceptible has "effective contact" with a specified case during one time period.

$(1-p)$ = probability that a susceptible fails to contact a specified case during one time period.

$(1-p)^{C_t}$ = probability that a susceptible fails to contact any of the C_t cases present during time period t.

$1-(1-p)^{C_t}$ = probability that a susceptible contacts at least one case during time period t.

= proportion of susceptibles present during time period (i.e. S_t) which have effective contact with at least one case during that time period.

Therefore:

$$C_{t+1} = S_t\{1-(1-p)^{C_t}\} \tag{A8}$$

which is the basic Reed-Frost equation (3).

D. Analogy between the mass-action and Reed-Frost formulations

The similarity between the mass-action and Reed-Frost models is illustrated as follows:

The basic mass-action equation (1), may be expressed as

$$\frac{C_{t+1}}{S_t} = C_t \cdot b \tag{A9}$$

The basic Reed-Frost equation (3,4) may likewise be expressed as

$$\frac{C_{t+1}}{S_t} = 1-(1-p)^{C_t} \tag{A10}$$

The right-hand side of this equation may be expanded, using the binomial theorem:

$$\frac{C_{t+1}}{S_t} = 1-(1-C_t p)+\frac{C_t(C_t-1)}{2!}p^2 - \frac{C_t(C_t-1)(C_t-2)p^3}{3!} + \cdots p^{C_t} \tag{A11}$$

If p, the probability of effective contact, is very small (say $p < 0.01$), then all the second degree or higher terms in this equation become negligible, and one is left with

$$\frac{C_{t+1}}{S_t} = 1 - 1 + C_t p = C_t p$$

which is identical to the mass-action equation (A9).

This demonstrates that, under conditions where the contact rate between any two specified individuals is small (as might occur in a very large *randomly* mixing population), then the mass-action and Reed-Frost models become effectively equivalent, and the epidemic threshold is then roughly the reciprocal of the probability of contact between individuals. This equivalence is intuitively reasonable, for with very low contact probabilities it becomes unlikely that any one susceptible would contact more than one case.

E. Chain binomial and Reed-Frost probability equations

In the chain binomial class of models, we consider there to be S_t susceptibles and C_t infectious cases at time t. Each of the susceptibles has an equal chance of becoming a case in the next time period, that chance being defined as a constant p^*, independent of C_t, in the Greenwood chain binomial, or as dependent on the number of cases, i.e. $\{1 - (1 - p)^{C_t}\}$ in the Reed-Frost model. The probability that any specified number of cases occurs in the next time period can then be expressed using the standard formula for binomial trials, i.e. for the Greenwood model:

$$\text{Prob}\ (C_{t+1} \mid C_t, S_t) = \frac{S_t!}{C_{t+1}!\, S_{t+1}!} p^{*C_t+1} (1 - p^*)^{S_t+1} \qquad \text{(A12)}$$

and for the Reed-Frost:

$$\text{Prob}\ (C_{t+1} \mid C_t, S_t) = \frac{S_t!}{C_{t+1}!\, S_{t+1}!} (1 - (1 - \text{p})^{C_t})^{C_{t+1}} \cdot (1 - p)^{C_t \cdot S_{t+1}} \qquad \text{(A13)}$$

These are discrete time, stochastic models, appropriate to describe the variation in courses of epidemics in small populations. Abbey (1952) and Bailey (1975) describe maximum likelihood methods for estimating p^* or p for any small epidemic or series of family epidemics.

F. The Rvachev-Baroyan geographic spread model

The Rvachev-Baroyan model for geographic spread of influenza appears in slightly different form in different publications. In general, it consists of the following sets of equations for each of n (typically $n = 128$) population centers considered: For city i:

$$dx_i/dt = \frac{-\beta_i}{P_i} x_i \int_0^\tau y_i \, g(\tau) \, d\tau + \sum_{j=1}^{n} \left(\frac{\sigma_{ji}}{P_j} x_j - \frac{\sigma_{ij}}{P_i} x_i \right) \qquad \text{(A14)}$$

$$dy_i/dt + dy_i/d\tau = \sum \left(\frac{\sigma_{ji}}{P_j} y_j - \frac{\sigma_{ij}}{P_i} y_i \right) \qquad \text{(A15)}$$

$$y_i(0, t) = \frac{\beta_i}{P_i} x_i \int_0^\tau y_i \, g(\tau) \, d\tau \qquad \text{(A16)}$$

where x and y are numbers of susceptibles and cases, and β is a transmission factor, as in Appendix B. The function $g(\tau)$ is the distribution of duration of cases similar to the function explored by Spicer (1979), in effect the W term in text equation 6, Section 2.4.1. The population of city i is P_i, and the rate of migration from city i to city j is called σ_{ij}. Equation A14 may be interpreted as stating that the change in number of susceptibles in city i, per unit time, is equal to the sum of susceptible immigrants from all cites, minus the sum of susceptible emigrants to all cities, minus the incidence of new infections in city i. Equation A15 is a partial derivative expression indicating that prevalence in city i is influenced by both in and out migration cases. And equation A16 is a continuous time version of the mass-action equation as used by Spicer (1979) – see text equation 6 in Section 2.4.1.

G. The Serfling regression model

Serfling's regression equation for weekly mortality in week t ($= M_t$) is often expressed as follows:

$$M_t = a + mt + f_1 \frac{\cos 2\pi t}{52} + h_1 \frac{\sin 2\pi t}{52} + f_2 \frac{\cos 4\pi t}{52} + h_2 \frac{\sin 4\pi t}{52} \qquad \text{(A17)}$$

where a is the average over the time period and m is the slope for linear trend. Houseworth and Langmuir (1974) added a second degree term for curvi-linear trend. The sin and cos terms are phrased so as to provide 6- and 12-month periodicity, giving a shape as illustrated in Figure 6A (p. 58).

5. Glossary of algebraic symbols

All algebraic symbols used in the text are defined briefly below. They are listed in the order in which they appear. The section in which they are introduced is given in parentheses.

t = Time (section 1.3.1).
In discrete time models, t, $t+1$, $t+2$ refer to successive time periods, each equivalent to a generation time (= serial interval) of influenza.

S = Number of susceptibles (section 2.1.1).
This often appears with a subscript, e.g. S_0, S_t, or S_{t+1}, indicating the time period to which reference is made.

C = Number of cases (section 2.1.1).
Subscripted as for susceptibles.

b = Transmission parameter used in simple discrete time mass-action equation (section 2.1.1).

β = Transmission parameter used in continuous time version of the mass-action equation (section 2.1.1).

x = Number of susceptibles in continuous time models (section 2.1.1).

y = Number of (infectious) cases in continuous time models (section 2.1.1).

z = Number of immunes in continuous time models (section 2.1.1).

p = "Probability of effective contact" (section 2.1.1).
This is the basic parameter of Reed-Frost-type models, and is generally defined as the "probability that any two individuals, selected at random from the population in question, have that sort of contact which is necessary for transmission of the infection, in one time period."

p^* = Probability that a susceptible individual becomes infected, during one time period (section 2.2).

This is the basic parameter of the Greenwood-type chain binomial models, and is equivalent to Hope-Simpson's (1952) "susceptible exposure attack rate".

p^*_i = Probability that a susceptible individual becomes infected by contact within the home (section 2.2).

p^*_e = Probability that a susceptible individual becomes infected by contact outside the home (section 2.2).

D = Duration of infectiousness of a case (section 2.3.1).
Use of this parameter implies an assumption of constant duration of infectiousness.

γ = Recovery rate in continuous time mass-action or Kermack-McKendrick type models (section 2.3.1 and Appendix B).

e = Base of natural logarithms (=2.718 ...).

W_T = Probability an individual remains infectious, T days after becoming infected (section 2.4.1).

α = Basic case transmission rate (section 2.4.1).
This describes the average number of effective contacts, or successful transmissions made by a single individual case in the early phase of an epidemic. Conceptually analogous to Macdonald's (1957) basic reproduction rate.

P = Total size of population considered (section 2.5.1).

r = Recovery rate in discrete time models (Appendix A).
This is the proportion of cases which recover (or are otherwise removed, as by dying) in one time period.

$g(\tau)$ = Function describing the duration of infectiousness of cases, analogous to W_T above (Appendix F).

M_t = Daily mortality from pneumonia and influenza, as "predicted" by Serfling's equation (Appendix G).

6. References

Note: References followed by a single asterisk were available only in part (e.g. as an English summary) for this review. References followed by two asterisks were not consulted at all.

Abbey, H. (1952) An examination of the Reed-Frost theory of epidemics, *Human Biol., 24,* 201-33.

Alling, D.W., Blackwelder, W.C., and Stuart-Harris, C. H. (1981) A study of excess mortality during influenza epidemics in the United States, 1968-1976, *Amer. J. Epid., 113,* 30-43.

Andrewes, C.H. (1951) The epidemiology of influenza in the light of the 1951 outbreak, *Proc. Roy. Soc. Med., 44,* 803-4.

Armitage, P. (1975) Epidemiology and statistics, *Bull. Int. Statist. Inst., 46,* 258-64.

Assaad, F., Cockburn, W.C., and Sundaresan, T.K. (1973) Use of excess mortality from respiratory diseases in the study of influenza, *Bull. Wld Hlth Org., 49,* 219-33.

Bailey, N.T.J. (1975) *The mathematical theory of infectious diseases and its applications,* London: Charles Griffin.

Bailey, N.T.J. (1980) Spatial models in the epidemiology of infectious diseases, *Lecture Notes in Biomathematics, 38,* 233-61.

Baroyan, O. V., Basilevsky, U. V., Ermakov, V. V., Frank, K. D., Rvachev, L. A., and Shashkov, V. A. (1970) Computer modelling of influenza epidemics for large-scale systems of cities and territories (working paper for WHO Symposium on Quantitative Epidemiology, Moscow, 23-27 November 1970 (in English and Russian).

Baroyan, O. V., Genchikov, L. A., Rvachev, L. A., and Shashkov, V. A. (1969) An attempt at large-scale influenza epidemic modelling by means of a computer, *Bull. Int. Epid. Assoc., 18,* 22-31.

Baroyan, O. V., and Rvachev, L. A. (1967) Deterministic epidemic models for a territory with a transport network, *Kibernetika, 3,* 67-74 (in Russian)**.

Baroyan, O. V., and Rvachev, L. A. (1968) Some epidemiological experiments carried out on an electronic computer, *Vestnik Akad. Med. Nauk, 23,* 32-4 (in Russian)**.

Baroyan, O. V., and Rvachev, L. A. (1977) *Mathematics and epidemiology,* Moscow: Znanie (in Russian).

Baroyan, O. V., Rvachev, L. A., Basilevsky, U. V., Ermakov, V. V., Frank, K. D., Rvachev, M. A., and Shashkov, V. A. (1971) Computer modelling of influenza epidemics for the whole country (USSR), *Adv. Appl. Prob., 3,* 224-26.

Baroyan, O V., Rvachev, L. A., Frank, K. D., Shashkov, V. A., and Basilevsky, U. V. (1973) Mathematical and computer modelling of influenza epidemics in the USSR, *Vestnik Akad. Med. Nauk, 28,* 26-30 (in Russian)**.

Baroyan, O. V., Rvachev, L. A., and Ivannikov, Yu. G. (1977) *Modelling and prediction of influenza epidemics in the USSR,* Moscow: N. F. Gamaleia Institute of Epidemiology and Microbiology (in Russian)*.

Baroyan, O. V., Zhdanov, V. M., Soloviev, V. D., Zakstelskaya, L. Ya., Rvachev, L. A., Urbakh, Yu. V., Ermakov, V. V., and Antonova, I. V. (1972) Prospects of machine modelling of influenza epidemics for the territory of the USSR, *Zh. Mikrobiol. Epidemiol. Immunobiol., 49,* 3-11 (in Russian)*.

Bartlett, M. S. (1960) The critical community size for measles in the United States, *J. Roy. Statist. Soc.,* Series A, *123,* 37-44.

Benenson, A. S., ed. (1975) *Control of communicable diseases in man* (12th edition), Washington, D.C.: Amer. Publ. Hlth Assoc.

Beveridge, W. I. B. (1977) *Influenza: the last great plague,* London: Heinemann.

Brownlee, J. (1915) Historical note on Farr's theory of the epidemic, *Brit. Med. J., ii,* 250-2.

Brownlee, J. (1919) The next epidemic of influenza, *Lancet, ii,* 856-7.

Brownlee, J. (1923) A further note upon the periodicity of influenza, *Lancet, i,* 1116.

Carey, D. E., Dunn, F. L., Robinson, R. Q., Jensen, K. E., and Martin, J. D. (1958) Community-wide epidemic of Asian strain influenza: clinical and subclinical illnesses among school children, *J. Amer. Med. Assoc., 167,* 1459-63.

Centers for Disease Control (1978) Reye syndrome—United States, *Morbidity and Mortality Weekly Reports,* vol. 27, pp. 15-16.

Chin, T. D. Y., Foley, J. F., Doto, I. L., Gravelle, C. R., and Weston, J. (1960) Morbidity and mortality characteristics of Asian strain influenza, *Publ. Hlth Rep., 75,* 149-58.

Choi, K. and Thacker, S. B. (1981) An evaluation of influenza mortality surveillance, 1962-1979: (I) Time series forecasts of expected pneumonia and influenza deaths, *Amer. J. Epid., 113,* 215-26.

Choi, K., and Thacker, S. B. (1981) An evaluation of influenza mortality surveillance, 1962-1979: (II) Percentage of pneumonia and influenza deaths as an indicator of influenza activity, *Amer. J. Epid., 113,* 227-35.

Cliff, A. D., Haggett, P., Ord, J. K., and Versey, G. R. (1981) *Spatial diffusion: an historical geography of measles epidemics in an island community,* Cambridge: Cambridge University Press.

Clifford, R. E., Smith, J. W. G., Tillett, H. E., and Wherry, P. J. (1977) Excess mortality associated with influenza in England and Wales, *Int. J. Epid., 6,* 115-28.

Collins, S. D. (1930) Influenza-pneumonia mortality in a group of about 95 cities in the United States, 1920-1929, *Publ. Hlth Rep., 45,* 361-406.

Collins, S. D. (1932) Excess mortality from causes other than influenza and pneumonia during influenza epidemics, *Publ. Hlth Rep., 47,* 2159-80.

Commission on Acute Respiratory Diseases (1946) The periodicity of influenza, *Amer. J. Hyg., 43,* 29-37.

Cristea, A. L., Petrescu, A. L., and Copelovici, Y. (1975) Utilisation d'un modèle mathématique de l'évolution de la morbidité par certaines viroses pour la caracterisation de l'épidémiologie de la grippe dans la R. S. de Roumanie. Note I, *Virologie, 26,* 87-97.

Cristea, A. L., Petrescu, A. L., Copelovici, Y., and Cajal, N. (1974), Utilization of mathematical processing of serograms in the survey of some aspects in influenza epidemiology, *Rev. Roum. Virol., 25,* 295-302.

Cristea, A., Petrescu, A., Copelovici, Y., Strulovica, D., Cajal, S. N., Dinca, A., Niculescu, R., Badescu, F., Puca, D., Zubac, I., Cretco, T., and Surianu, C. (1976) Utilisation d'un modèle mathématique de l'évolution de la morbidité par certaines viroses pour la caracterisation de l'épidémiologie de la grippe dans la R. S. de Roumanie. Note II. Analyse de l'épidémiologie de la grippe dans une zone géographique à morbidité élevée, *Virologie, 27,* 13-25.

Damms, V. G. S., Clarke, A. H., and Constable, G. M. (1976) A mathematical approach to epidemic control, *J. Roy. Coll. Gen. Pract., 26,* 911-6.

Davey, M. L., and Reid, D. (1972) Relationship of air temperature to outbreaks of influenza, *Brit. J. Prev. Soc. Med., 26,* 28-32.

Davis, L. E., Caldwell, G. G., Lynch, R. E., Bailey, R. F., and Chin, T. D. Y. (1970) Hong Kong influenza: the epidemiologic features of a high school family study analyzed and compared with a similar study during the 1957 Asian influenza epidemic, *Amer. J. Epid., 92,* 240-7.

Dowdle, W. R., Coleman, M. T., and Gregg, M. B. (1974) Natural history of influenza type A in the United States, 1957-1972, *Progr. med. Virol., 17,*91-135.

Dunn, F. L., Carey, D. E., Cohen, A., and Martin, J. D. (1959) Epidemiologic studies of Asian influenza in a Louisiana parish, *Amer. J. Hyg., 70,* 351-71.

Eickhoff, T. C., Sherman, I. L., and Serfling, R. E. (1961) Observations on excess mortality associated with epidemic influenza, *J. Amer. Med. Assoc., 176,* 776-82.

Elveback, L. (1971) Simulation of stochastic discrete time epidemic models for two agents, *Adv. Appl. Prob., 3,* 231-2.

Elveback, L., Ackerman, E., Gatewood, L., and Fox, J. P. (1971) Stochastic two-agent epidemic simulation models for a community of families, *Amer. J. Epid., 93,* 267-80.

Elveback, L. R., Ackerman, E., Young, G., and Fox, J. P. (1968) A stochastic model for competition between viral agents in the presence of interference. 1. Live virus vaccine in a randomly mixing population, Model III, *Amer. J. Epid., 87,* 373-84.

Elveback, L., Fox, J. P., and Ackerman, E. (1975) Simulation models (Proceedings of the 40th session of the International Statistical Institute), *I.S.I. Bulletin,* vol. 46, book 1, pp. 553-68.

Elveback, L. R., Fox, J. P., Ackerman, E., Langworthy, A., Boyd, M., and Gatewood, L. (1976) An influenza simulation model for immunization studies, *Amer. J. Epid., 103,* 152-65.

Elveback, L. R., Fox, J. P., and Ackerman, E. (1976) Stochastic simulation models for two immunization problems, *SIAM Review, 18,* 52-61.

Elveback, L., Fox, J. P., and Varma, A. (1964) An extension of the Reed-Frost epidemic model for the study of competition between viral agents in the presence of interference, *Amer. J. Hyg., 80,* 356-64.

Evans, G. H. (1876) Some arithmetical considerations of the progress of epidemics, *Trans. Epid. Soc., 3,* 551-55.

Ewy, W., Ackerman, E., Gatewood, L. C., Elveback, L., and Fox, J. P. (1972) A generalized stochastic model for simulation of epidemics in a heterogeneous population (Model VI), *Comput. Biol. Med., 2,* 45-58.

Farr, W. (1847) *Tenth annual report of the Registrar General,* London: HMSO.

Farr, W. (1866) On the cattle plague (Letter to Editor of the Daily News, London), 19 February 1866.

Fazekas de St. Groth, S. (1975) Influenza: antigenic evolution and epidemiology, *Bull. Int. Statist. Inst., 66* (1), 467-77.

Fine, P. E. M. (1975) Ross's a priori pathometry—a perspective, *Proc. Roy. Soc. Med., 68,* 547-51.

Fine, P. E. M. (1977) A commentary on the mechanical analogue to the Reed-Frost model, *Amer. J. Epid., 106,* 87-100.

Fine, P. E. M. (1979) John Brownlee and the measurement of infectiousness: an historical study in epidemic theory, *J. Roy. Statist. Soc.,* Series A, *142,* 347-62.

Fortmann, A. (1976) Abstract model and epidemiological reality of influenza A, in: Berger, J. et al., eds., *Mathematical models in medicine,* Vol. 11, pp. 58-73, Berlin: Springer.

Fortmann, A., and Florin, H. (1975) Die Ausbreitung der Influenza A—Versuch der Simulation durch ein mathematisches Modell (Spreading of influenza A—simulation through a mathematical model), *Öff. Gesundheitswes., 37,* 318-31.

Fox, J. P., Elveback, L., Scott, W., Gatewood, L., and Ackerman, E. (1971) Herd immunity: basic concept and relevance to public health immunization practices, *Amer. J. Epid., 94,* 179-89.

Fox, J. P., and Kilbourne, E. D., rapporteurs (1973) From the National Institutes of Health: Epidemiology of influenza—summary of influenza workshop IV, *J. Inf. Dis., 128,* 361-86.

Francis, T., Magill, T. P., Rickard, E. R., and Beck, M. D. (1937) Etiological and serological studies in epidemic influenza, *Amer. J. Publ. Hlth, 27,* 1141-60.

Frost, W. H. (1976) Some conceptions of epidemics in general, *Amer. J. Epid., 103,* 141-51.

Gatewood, L. C. (1971) Stochastic simulation of influenza A epidemics within a structured community (Ph.D. dissertation), University of Minnesota**.

Greenwood, M. (1931) On the statistical measure of infectiousness, *J. Hyg. (Camb.), 31,* 336-51.

Greenwood, M. (1949) The infectiousness of measles, *Biometrika, 36,* 1-8.

Gregg, M. B., Bregman, D. J., O'Brien, R. J., and Millar, J. D. (1978) Influenza-related mortality, *J. Amer. Med. Assoc., 239,* 115-16.

Hamer, W. H. (1906) Epidemic disease in England, *Lancet, i,* 733-39.

Hammond, B. J. and Tyrrell, D. A. J. (1971) A mathematical model of common cold epidemics on Tristan da Cunha, *J. Hyg. (Camb.), 69,* 423-33.

Hattis, R. P., Halstead, S. B., Herrmann, K. L., and Witte, J. J. (1973) Rubella in an immunized island population, *J. Amer. Med. Assoc., 223,* 1019-21.

Heasman, M. A., and Reid, D. D. (1961) Theory and observation in family epidemics of the common cold, *Brit. J. Prev. Soc. Med., 15,* 12-16.

Henderson, D. A. (1972) Epidemiology in the global eradication of smallpox, *Int. J. Epid., 1,* 25-30.

Hope Simpson, R. E. (1948) The period of transmission in certain epidemic diseases, *Lancet, ii,* 755-60.

Hope Simpson, R. E. (1952) Infectiousness of communicable diseases in the household, *Lancet, ii,* 549-54.

Hope Simpson, R. E. (1958) Discussion on the common cold, *Proc. Roy. Soc. Med., 51,* 267-71.

Hope Simpson, R. E. (1970) First outbreak of Hong Kong influenza in a general practice population in Great Britain. A field and laboratory study, *Brit. Med. J., 3,* 74-7.

Hope Simpson, R. E. (1978) Sunspots and flu: a correlation, *Nature, 275,* 86.

Hope Simpson, R. E. (1979) Epidemic mechanisms of type A influenza, *J. Hyg. (Camb.), 83,* 11-26.

Hope Simpson, R.E. and Sutherland, I. (1954) Does influenza spread within the household?, *Lancet, i,* 721-26.

Houseworth, J., and Langmuir, A. D. (1974) Excess mortality from epidemic influenza, *Amer. J. Epid., 100,* 40-8.

Houseworth, W.J. and Spoon, M. M. (1971) The age distribution of excess mortality during A2 Hong Kong influenza epidemics compared with earlier A2 outbreaks, *Amer. J. Epid., 94,* 348-50.

Hoyle, F. and Wickramasinghe, C. (1979) *Diseases from space,* London: Dent.

Ipsen, J. (1959) Social distance in epidemiology—age of susceptible siblings as the determining factor in household infectivity of measles, *Human Biology, 31,* 162-79.

Isaacs, A. and Andrewes, C. H. (1951) The spread of influenza. Evidence from 1950-1951, *Brit. Med. J., 2,* 921-27.

Jordan, W.S., Denny, F.W., Badger, C.C., Dingle, J.H., Oseasohn, R., and Stevens, D.A. (1958) A study of illness in a group of Cleveland families, *Amer. J. Hyg., 68,* 190-212.

Kemper, J. T. (1980) Error sources in the evaluation of secondary attack rates, *Amer. J. Epid., 112,* 457-66.

Kendal, A. P., Schieble, J., Cooney, M. K., Chin, J., Foy, H. M., and Noble, G. R. (1978) Co-circulation of two influenza A (H_3N_2) antigenic variants detected by virus surveillance in individual communities, *Amer. J. Epid., 108,* 308-11.

Kermack, W. O., and McKendrick, A. G. (1927) Contributions to the mathematical theory of epidemics, Part I, *Proc. Roy. Soc., A 115,* 700-21.

Kilbourne, E. D. (1978) Influenza mortality and morbidity, *J. Amer. Med. Assoc., 239,* 107.

Langmuir, A. D. (1976) William Farr: Founder of modern concepts of surveillance, *Int. J. Epid., 5,* 13-18.

Langmuir, A. D. (1977) A re-examination of herd immunity (Heath Clark lectures, delivered at London School of Hygiene and Tropical Medicine) (to be published).

Lidwell, O. M., and Somerville, J. (1951) Observations on the incidence and distribution of the common cold in a rural community during 1948 and 1949, *J. Hyg. (Camb.), 49,* 365-81.

Longini, I. M. (1977) Optimal control of influenza A epidemics (Ph.D. dissertation), University of Minnesota.**

Longini, I. M., Ackerman, G., and Elveback, L. R. (1978) An optimization model for influenza A epidemics, *Math. Biosciences, 38,* 141-57.

Loosli, C. G., Robertson, O. H., and Puck, T. T. (1943a) The production of experimental influenza in mice by inhalation of atmospheres containing influenza virus dispersed as fine droplets, *J. infect. Dis., 72,* 142-53.

Loosli, C. G., Lemon, H. M., Robertson, O. H., and Appel, E. (1943b) Experimental air-borne influenza infection. I. Influence of humidity on survival of virus in air, *Proc. Soc. Exp. Biol. Med., 53,* 205-6.

MacDonald, G. (1957) *The epidemiology and control of malaria,* Oxford: Oxford University Press.

Mantle, J., and Tyrrell, D. A. J. (1973) An epidemic of influenza on Tristan da Cunha, *J. Hyg. (Lond.), 71,* 89-95.

Masurel, N. (1976) Swine influenza virus and the recycling of influenza A viruses in man, *Lancet, ii,* 244-47.

Mau-Lang, W. (1979) Dual recombination as origin of pandemic influenza viruses, *Lancet, ii,* 1077.

McFarlane, A. (1976) Daily mortality and environment in English conurbations. I. Air pollution, low temperature, and influenza in Greater London, *Brit. J. Prev. Soc. Med., 31,* 54-61.

Monto, A. S., Davenport, F. M., Napier, J. A., and Francis, T. (1969) Effect of vaccination of a school age population upon the course of an A2/Hong Kong influenza epidemic, *Bull. Wld Hlth Org., 41,* 537-42.

Moser, M. R., Bender, T. R., Margolis, H. S., Noble, G. R., Kendal, A. P., and Ritter, D. G. (1979) An outbreak of influenza aboard a commercial airliner, *Amer. J. Epid., 110,* 1-6.

Muench, H. (1959) *Catalytic models in epidemiology,* Cambridge, Mass.: Harvard University Press.

Nakajima, K., Desselberger, V., and Palese, F. (1978) Recent human influenza A (H_1N_1) viruses are closely related genetically to strains isolated in 1950, *Nature, 274,* 334-39.

Neustadt, R. E., and Fineberg, H. V. (1978) *The swine flu affair: Decision-making on a slippery disease,* Washington, D.C.: US Government Printing Office.

Owada, K., Sakamoto, K., and Tanaka, H. (1971) An epidemiological study on incubation period of influenza, *Jap. J. Hyg., 26,* 264-67.

Peretjagina, N. S., Antonova, I. V., and Urbah, V. Ju. (1977) The upper tolerance limits of non-epidemic daily morbidity for influenza and other acute respiratory diseases in the epidemic season, *Bull. Wld Hlth Org., 55,* 761-63.

Retailliau, H. F., Storch, G. A., Curtis, A. C., Horne, T. J., Scally, M. J., and Hattwick, M. A. W. (1979) The epidemiology of influenza B in a rural setting in 1977, *Amer. J. Epid., 109,* 639-49.

Rickard, E. R., Lennette, E. H., and Horsfall, F. L. (1940) Comprehensive study of influenza in a rural community, *Publ. Hlth Rep., 55,* 2146-67.

Ross, R. (1915) Some *a priori* pathometric equations, *Brit. Med. J., 1,* 546-47.

Rvachev, L. A. (1967) A model for the connection between processes in the organism and the structure of epidemics, *Kibernetika, 3,* 75-8 (in Russian)**.

Rvachev, L. A. (1968) Computer modelling experiment on large scale epidemics, *Dokl. Akad. Nauk SSSR,* vol. 180, no. 2, pp. 294-96.

Rvachev, L. A. (1968) Modelling of the connection between epidemiological and infectious processes, *Vestnik Akad. Med. Nauk,* vol. 23, no. 5, pp. 34-9 (in Russian)**.

Rvachev, L. A. (1971) A computer experiment for predicting an influenza epidemic, *Dokl. Akad. Nauk SSSR,* vol. 198, no. 1, pp. 68-70 (in Russian).

Rvachev, L. A. (1972) Modelling medico-biological processes in a community in terms of the dynamics of continuous media, *Dokl. Akad. Nauk SSSR,* vol. 203, no. 3, pp. 540-42 (in Russian)**.

Sabin, A. B. (1977) Mortality from pneumonia and risk conditions during influenza epidemics. High influenza morbidity during nonepidemic years, *J. Amer. Med. Assoc., 237,* 2823-28.

Salk, J. E., Menke, W. J., and Francis, T. (1945) Clinical epidemiological and immunological evaluation of vaccine against epidemic influenza, *Amer. J. Hyg., 42,* 57-93.

Sartwell, P. (1950) The distribution of incubation periods of infectious disease, *Amer. J. Hyg., 51,* 310-18.

Schild, G. C., Newman, R. W., McGregor, I. A., and Williams, K. (1977) The use of transportable single-radial-diffusion immunoplates in seroepidemiological studies of influenza in The Gambia, *Bull. Wld Hlth Org., 55,* 3-13.

Schulman, J. L., and Kilbourne, E. D. (1963) Experimental transmission of influenza virus infection in mice. II. Some factors affecting the incidence of transmitted infection, *J. Exp. Med., 118,* 267-75.

Selby, P., ed. (1976) *Influenza: virus, vaccines, and strategy* (Proceedings of a working group on pandemic influenza, Rougemont, 26-28 January 1976), London and New York: Academic Press.

Serfling, R. E. (1963) Methods for current statistical analysis of excess pneumonia-influenza deaths, *Publ. Hlth Rep., 78,* 494-506.

Serfling, R. E., Sherman, I. L., and Houseworth, W. J. (1967) Excess pneumonia-influenza mortality by age and sex in three major influenza A2 epidemics, United States, 1957-58, 1960, and 1963, *Amer. J. Epid., 86,* 433-41.

Shope, R. E. (1936) The incidence of neutralizing antibodies for swine influenza virus in the sera of human beings of different ages, *J. Exp. Med., 63,* 669-84.

Smith, J. W. G. (1976) Vaccination strategy, in: Selby, P., ed., *Influenza: virus, vaccines, and strategy* (Proceedings of a working group on pandemic influenza, Rougemont, 26-28 January 1976), London and New York: Academic Press.

Soper, H. E. (1929) Interpretation of periodicity in disease prevalence, *J. Roy. Statist. Soc., 92,* 34-73.

Spicer, C. C. (1979) The mathematical modelling of influenza epidemics, *Brit. Med. Bull., 35,* 23-8.

Stuart-Harris, C. H. and Schild, G. C. (1976) *Influenza: the viruses and the disease*, London: Edward Arnold.

Sugiyama, H. (1960) Some statistical contributions to the health sciences, *Osaka City Medical Journal, 6,* 141-58.

Sugiyama, H. (1961) Some statistical methodologies for epidemiological research of medical sciences, *Bull. Int. Statist. Inst.,* vol. 38, no. 3, pp. 137-51.

Tillett, H. E., Smith, J. W. G., and Clifford, R. E. (1980) Excess morbidity and mortality associated with influenza in England and Wales, *Lancet, i,* 793-95.

Webster, R. G., Campbell, C. H., and Granoff, A. (1973) The *in vivo* production of "new" influenza A viruses. III. Isolation of recombinant influenza viruses under simulated conditions of natural transmission, *Virology, 51,* 149-62.

Wilson, E. B., Bennett, C., Allen, M., and Worcester, J. (1939) Measles and scarlet fever in Providence, R. I., 1929-34 with respect to age and size of family, *Proc. Amer. Phil. Soc., 80,* 357-476.

World Health Organization (1979) Influenza in the world: October 1977-September 1978, *Wkly epidem. Rec., 54,* 25-8.

World Health Organization (1980) Influenza in the world: October 1978-September 1979, *Wkly epidem. Rec., 55,* 17-20.

World Health Organization (1980) Influenza nomenclature, *Wkly epidem. Rec., 55,* 294-95.

Wright, P. F., Thompson, J., and Karzon, D. T. (1980) Differing virulence of H_1N_1 and H_3N_2 influenza strains, *Amer. J. Epid., 112,* 814-19.

Yamamoto, K. (1959) A theoretical epidemiological study on the mode of infection of influenza in the household, *J. Osaka City Med. Center, 9,* 2179-90.

Yorke, J. A., Nathanson, N., Pianigiani, G., and Martin, J. (1979) Seasonality and the requirements for perpetuation and eradication of viruses in populations, *Amer. J. Epid., 109,* 103-23.

Session I

The epidemiology of influenza–key facts and remaining problems

Stuart-Harris

J. Smith

The epidemiology of influenza: key facts and remaining problems (1)

C. H. Stuart-Harris

ABSTRACT

The basic characters of influenza epidemics are determined by the interplay between the viruses and their human hosts. The key features of periodicity, pandemicity, and variation in incidence are discussed in relation to changes in viral antigens and human serological changes.

The making of models of epidemic situations demands an appreciation of the behavior of such epidemics under natural conditions. It is, therefore, appropriate in this introduction briefly to review the key features concerning the epidemiology of influenza by referring in turn to periodicity, pandemicity, and the variation of the incidence of influenza from place to place and from one epidemic to the next.

Periodicity

Figure 1 shows the experience in England and Wales of influenza as a cause of death, for the years 1940 to 1970. The British practice of referring to "deaths from influenza" consists of adding together all death certificates on which influenza is mentioned as either a primary or a contributory cause of death. Such practice has been shown to produce a faithful though not exact index of influenza virus infection, when the weekly numbers of deaths are compared with the weekly numbers of laboratory isolations of viruses. But in Figure 1 it is the variation in magnitude of the epidemics which needs an explanation, and I hope to show for this that antigenic variation of the causative viruses is an important factor.

In 1940, the epidemic which occurred in England and Wales yielded many negative results in the laboratory. In New York City, however, the late Thomas Francis (1940) and T. P. Magill (1940) independently succeeded in recovering the first strains of influenza B in ferrets, and it is likely that the British epidemic was due to this virus. Then in 1943 there was a sharp epidemic of influenza A, the virus of which differed antigenically from the A viruses recovered first in 1932-33 in London, and then in Britain, the USA, and elsewhere in 1936-37. This

FIGURE 1

Influenza death rate per million, England and Wales, 1940-70

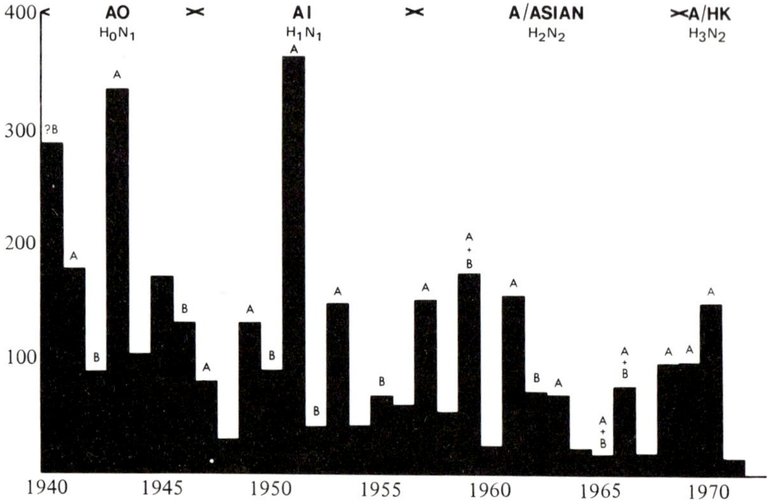

The figure shows the viruses concerned annually and the prevalent influenza A sub-types. From Stuart-Harris and Schild (1976).

1943 virus (Salk et al., 1944) became the first considerable variant since the viruses of the earlier years, and it probably arose by the step-by-step process now termed "drift". All the viruses of the outbreaks from 1932 to 1943 nevertheless remained in the sub-type described by the surface antigens, haemagglutinin and neuraminidase, as H_0N_1.

In 1951, the most lethal epidemic of the entire period shown in Figure 1 was associated with a rate which was, for some unknown reason, especially high in Liverpool, where the number of deaths equalled that in the 1918-19 pandemic. Hospitals were over-full, and the outbreak caused so much illness among nurses that wards had to be closed. The influenza A virus which caused this epidemic was of a new sub-type, H_1N_1, now regarded as a derivative of H_0N_1. This virus first appeared in Australia in 1946, it then appeared in 1947 in Britain and the USA, and a large epidemic occurred in Europe during the winter of 1948-49. From 1951 until 1957 influenza epidemics came and went throughout the world, their progress being monitored by the newly organized laboratory network of WHO.

In 1957 the first major antigenic shift occurred in the influenza A virus. An outbreak of influenza began in the south-eastern region of

China and spread rapidly to Malaysia, Japan, other adjoining countries, and ultimately the whole world (Langmuir, 1961; Payne, 1958). It seemed that introduction of the virus into tropical areas led immediately to explosive outbreaks. The Asian virus reached England and Wales and the USA in July 1957, but did not cause an epidemic until September and October. Figure 2 shows the form of the outbreaks derived from

FIGURE 2

Pneumonia notifications, England and Wales, 1957-59. Influenza A/Asian/57 (H_2N_2)

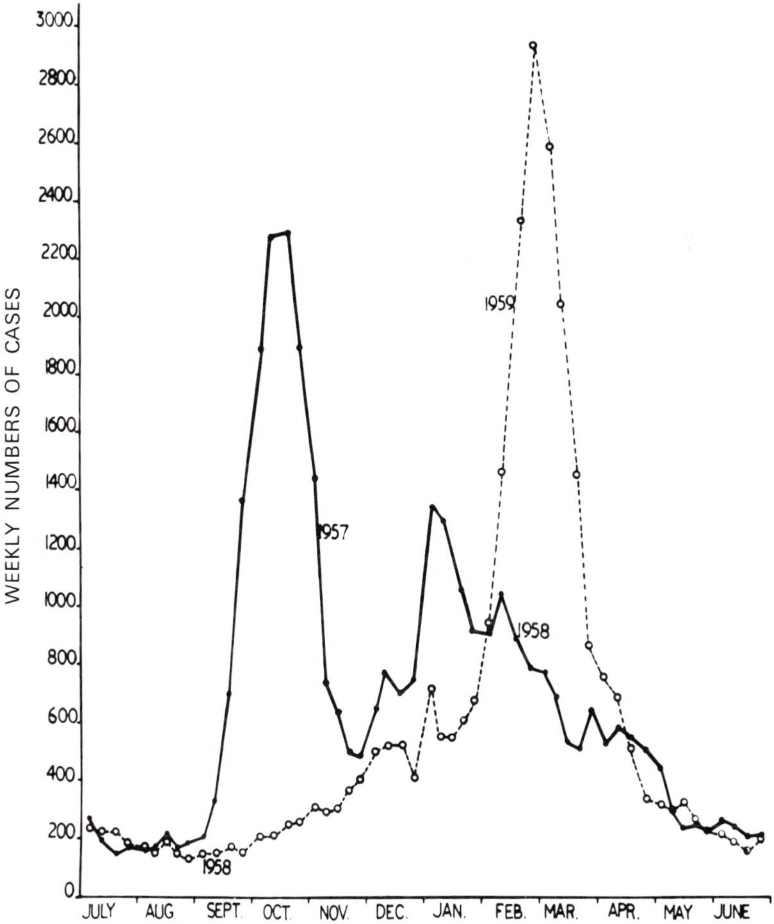

Reproduced by courtesy of the Department of Health and Social Security.

notifications of pneumonia in three waves: in 1957, in the early weeks of 1958, and in the winter of 1959-60. Deaths in the first few weeks of the 1957 outbreak were fewer than expected. The incidence in the population as a whole was 20-30%, the highest rate being in children aged 5-15 years. There were more deaths in the second outbreak in 1958, attributed to the virus spreading into older age groups. A relatively high mortality also occurred in 1959-60, although in that year influenza B also occurred in children.

Throughout the progress of the Asian pandemic deaths were primarily in persons over 60 years of age, unlike those in the 1918-19 pandemic which mainly involved those aged 20 to 40 years. The A/Asian (H_2N_2) virus maintained its surface antigens unchanged until after 1960; antigenic drift then occurred and continued until 1967-68, when the virus disappeared. At this time a new virus, A/Hong Kong/68, first appeared in China and began to spread like the Asian virus, though with less intensity (Cockburn et al., 1969). This virus had a new haemagglutinin (H_3) not encountered previously, and the same neuraminidase (N_2) as the Asian virus. In 1968, the first epidemic due to H_3N_2 virus was prolonged and grumbling in England and Wales, though the virus caused an explosive epidemic in the USA. In 1969-70, however, there occurred the largest outbreak in England and Wales for the past 12 years (Stuart-Harris, 1970). Figure 3 shows the curves of influenza deaths in 1932-33 and 1969-70. Although the viruses causing these outbreaks were unrelated in their surface antigens, their epidemic curves showed an equally rapid increase in mortality, and an equally rapid decrease after their peaks. Only the duration of the epidemic was different, the A/Hong Kong/68 epidemic ending more rapidly. The virus of this epidemic remained antigenically unchanged until 1972. Antigenic drift then occurred, and has continued at intervals ever since.

This brief survey of epidemics does not immediately suggest a close relationship between antigenic variation and death from influenza. However, mortality alone may not be the best index of influenza virus activity, and in Britain we appear to have an excellent index of morbidity. An examination of the recorded morbidity from influenza in the winter months from 1968 to 1977, reported weekly by a panel of GPs to the epidemic observation unit of the Royal College of General Practitioners, is shown in Figure 4 and Table 1. These also show total respiratory deaths each month from influenza, bronchitis, and influenzal pneumonia in England and Wales during the seven winter months from October to April. The viruses found each year by the Public Health Laboratory Service for England and Wales are also noted.

It must be borne in mind that the number of notifications refers to influenza in a population of about 150,000, whereas the deaths refer to

FIGURE 3

Comparison of influenza deaths in 1932-33 and 1969-70

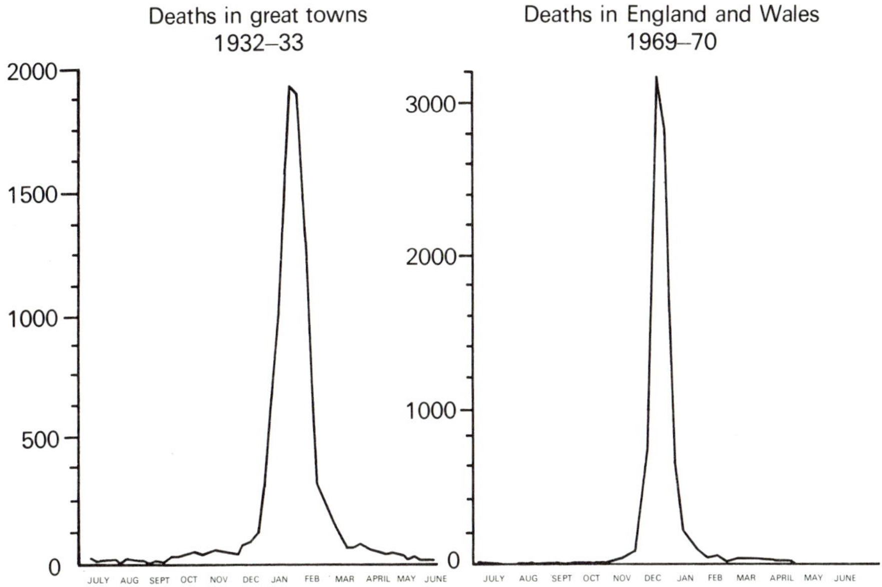

The left-hand curve shows the weekly numbers of deaths in the great towns (population 500,000 or over), which include about half the population of England and Wales, in 1932-33. The right-hand curve shows the weekly numbers of deaths in England and Wales, in 1969-70.

the total population of England and Wales, and to deaths from influenza, bronchitis, and influenzal pneumonia. This explains why the number of deaths is greater than the number of notifications.

The large swings in notifications for 1968-69, 1969-70, and 1971-72 represent the three A/Hong Kong epidemics. But the peaks in 1972-73 and 1975-76 are associated with the antigenic variants of A/England/72 and A/Victoria/75, respectively. In between these peaks are the ripples associated with the A/Port Chalmers/73 virus, which made little impact on the population. The H_3N_2 virus of 1977 (A/Texas/77) and the newly-arrived, recurrent H_1N_1 virus (A/USSR/77) caused little increase in mortality, though morbidity rose sharply. The morbidity/mortality ratio for each of the years in Table 1 indicates clearly the variation in severity of all these epidemics. For example, the ratio in 1970-71, a year with minimal influenza, was one notification to every 338 deaths, in contrast to the years with large

FIGURE 4

Comparison of morbidity and mortality in ten winter periods of the A/Hong Kong/68 era, 1968-78

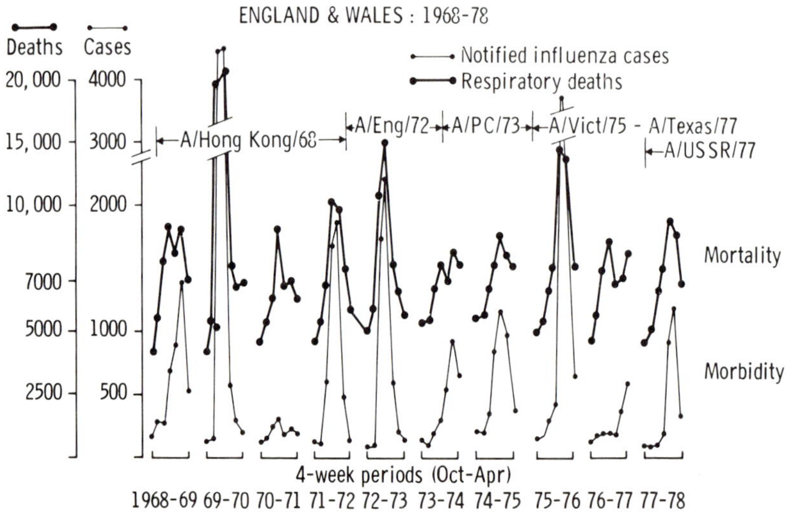

The figure shows the prevalence of the various viral strains during this period of antigenic drift. Notified influenza cases: information received by the epidemiological unit of the Royal College of General Practitioners, for October to April inclusive (actual numbers $\times$ 10). Respiratory deaths: deaths from influenza, bronchitis, and influenzal pneumonia, in October to April inclusive.

outbreaks of influenza when the ratios were approximately one in a hundred. Antigenically novel viruses, such as A/Hong Kong/68 and its derivatives, had a striking effect on both morbidity and mortality. A look at the impact of antigenic variants on the population, by estimating the proportion whose sera contained antibodies, confirmed this view. Antigenic variation is followed, year by year, by changes in the proportion of positive sera.

Tables 2 and 3 show the results of annual screening of sera collected each summer in Sheffield, from persons of all ages, arranged in decades. Table 2 shows the annual results, expressed as the proportion of sera for each age group with antibodies, estimated by the haemagglutination-inhibition test using the A/Hong Kong/68 virus. The increase in the proportion of sera with antibodies, after each of the three epidemics in 1968-69, 1969-70, and 1971-72, is obvious; 73-96% contained antibodies when this virus disappeared in 1972 and was replaced by

A/Eng/72. Table 3 continues the story with the three antigenic variants during epidemics from 1972-73 to 1975-76. The low proportion of sera with antibody to the A/Vict/75 virus in the summer of 1975 correlated well with the high morbidity experienced in the succeeding winter of 1975-76. There is some justification for regarding antigenic variation as a significant factor in the periodicity of influenza. This should be borne in mind when attempting to make predictions.

Nevertheless, the impact on the population of different pandemic viruses derived by antigenic shift is not exactly the same. Table 4 shows the attack rate calculated from sera collected randomly in 1957, after the first wave of Asian (H_2N_2) influenza, and in 1969, after the first wave in the winter of 1968-69 of A/Hong Kong (H_3N_2) virus. Whereas 50-70% of children and adolescents were sero-positive after the intensive attack of the Asian virus, the figure for the Hong Kong first epidemic was only about 30% in the same age groups.

TABLE 1

Relationship of influenza morbidity to total deaths from respiratory causes, in ten winter periods in England and Wales, 1968-78

Winter months Oct-April	*Influenza morbidity (index)*	*Respiratory deaths*	*Ratio of influenza mortality*	*Influenza A viruses*
1968-69	417.5	50,984	1:122	A/Hong Kong/68
1969-70	1,044.3	71,038	1:68	
1970-71	133.7	45,225	1:338	
1971-72	492.4	49,939	1:101	
1972-73	519.7	56,648	1:109	A/Eng/72
1973-74	273.3	47,714	1:174	A/PC/73
1974-75	401.8	49,563	1:123	
1975-76	772.1	60,138	1:78	A/Vict/75
1976-77	165.5	47,912	1:289	
1977-78	278.1	48,398	1:178	A/Texas/77 A/USSR/77

Influenza morbidity: information received by the epidemiological unit of the Royal College of General Practitioners, for October to April inclusive.

Respiratory deaths: deaths from influenza, bronchitis, and influenzal pneumonia, October to April inclusive.

Rank order of ratio by year: 69-70, 75-76, 71-72, 72-73, 68-69, 74-75, $\frac{73\text{-}74}{77\text{-}78}$, 76-77, 70-71.

TABLE 2

Haemagglutination-inhibition test for antibody to A/Hong Kong/68 virus, in sera collected annually in Sheffield

Age group	*Year of collection*					
	1968	*1969*	*1970*	*1971*	*1972*	*1973*
	Pre-epidemic	Post 1st epidemic	Post 2nd epidemic	—	Post 3rd epidemic	Change to A/Eng/42/72
0- 9	0	32	72	45	84	63
10-19	2	41	77	61	82	100
20-29	15	37	92	62	94	92
30-39	7	36	79	53	96	79
40-49	10	33	84	58	84	78
50-59	9	28	82	54	83	80
60-69	14	20	64	56	74	63
70-79	19	24	57	47	73	77
80 +	100	86	90	61	90	81

Sera were collected at random in summer each year. Numbers are percentages of sera with antibody, at 1:10 dilution, by age group. The table shows the rise in percentages of sera with antibody after each of three epidemics.

TABLE 3

Haemagglutination-inhibition test for antibody to the antigenic variants of A/Hong Kong/68 virus, in sera collected annually in Sheffield

Age group	*A/Eng/42/72*			*A/Port Chalmers/1/73*			*A/Vict/3/75*		
	1972	*1973*	*1974*	*1973*	*1974*	*1975*	*1975*	*1976*	*1977*
	Pre-epidemic	1st epidemic		Pre-epidemic	Post 1st epidemic	Post 2nd epidemic	Pre-epidemic	Post 1st epidemic	Post 2nd epidemic
0-9	70	65	57	41	63	33	22	75	44
10-19	70	79	70	29	50	89	7	26	84
20-29	76	73	58	31	27	52	12	86	70
30-39	52	60	23	54	23	52	0	42	59
40-49	55	56	62	37	21	58	18	78	40
50-59	48	63	80	66	27	50	26	58	72
60-69	54	57	87	48	43	31	8	70	56
70-79	42	77	73	67	32	38	25	70	36
80-89	40	75	37	78	12	51	36	63	32

Numbers are percentages of sera with antibody, at 1:10 dilution, by age group. The table shows the changes in percentages of sera with antibody to the particular strain of virus after epidemics in 1973, 1974, 1975, 1976, and 1977 (post-epidemic sera).

TABLE 4

Comparision of attack rates in 1957 and 1969, estimated from sera collected in Sheffield

Age group	*1957 (A/Sing/57)*	*1969 (A/Hong Kong/68)*
0-9	52	30
10-19	71	31
20-29	43	25
30-39	36	29
40-49	56	21.5
50-59	34	18.5
60-69	6	8
70-79	35	6
80 and over	47	0

Numbers are percentages, calculated by subtracting the percentage with antibody before the epidemic from the percentage with antibody to the homologous virus after the epidemic. From Stuart-Harris (1970).

Pandemicity

A look at the experience of England and Wales from 1850 to 1940 (Figure 5) shows the striking effect upon influenza deaths of two large pandemics. The first occurred in 1890-92, immediately after an unprecedented absence of mortality for 40 years (although some outbreaks have been described during this period). From an origin in central Asia in 1889, influenza spread westward to involve Europe fairly rapidly in 1890. Two further waves, with higher mortality, occurred in 1891 and 1892. The second pandemic, in 1918-19, caused an enormous mortality in all parts of the world, a large proportion of deaths occurring in those aged 20 to 40 years. There are many theories, but no completely satisfactory explanation, of the age distribution of this mortality. The pandemic started simultaneously in Europe and on the east coast of the USA. Each pandemic took the form of three separate waves, the first of which, though extensive, caused far fewer deaths than the other two. This is somewhat similar to the Asian pandemic of 1957. On the other hand, there is a close resemblance between the 1968-71 A/Hong Kong epidemics and the 1890-92 epidemics, but the Hong Kong virus caused far fewer deaths than the earlier pandemic.

Pandemics are characterized by their geographic spread and by the rapid increase in mortality which they produce. The Asian epidemic (Figure 6) was the first pandemic to be studied virologically, and its origin

FIGURE 5

Influenza death rate per million, England and Wales, 1850-1940

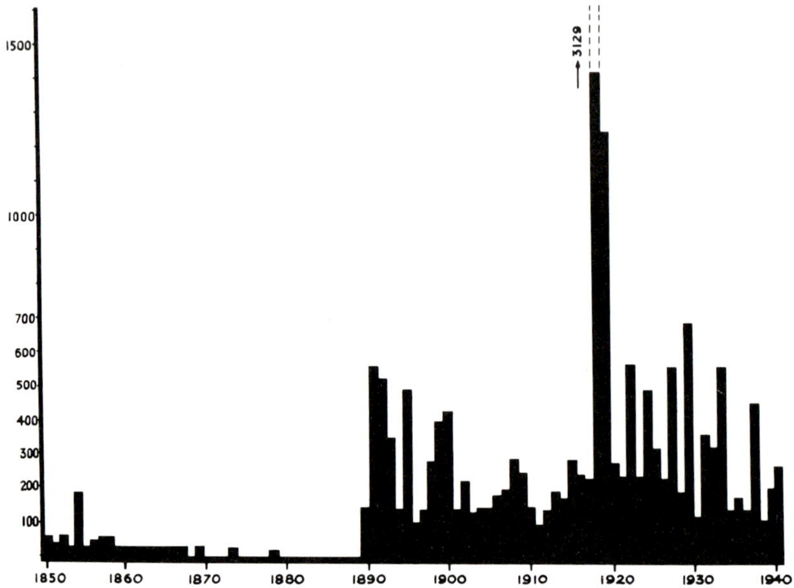

From Stuart-Harris and Schild (1976).

was certainly in south-east China. Outbreaks spread throughout south-east Asia and were documented month by month on their way to Europe. The pace of spread did not appear to be any greater than in previous pandemics, despite the increase in air traffic.

So far, virologists have only the Asian and Hong Kong viruses to study in seeking to understand pandemics. In each case a new antigenic sub-type of virus, with a previously unknown haemagglutinin, was able to roam over a human respiratory tract which had no specific humoral defence resulting from past infection. Serological analysis of people born before 1890 suggests that the virus of that year may share antigenic properties with the A/Hong Kong virus of 1968 (Masurel, 1969). There is also both serological and circumstantial evidence that the virus of the 1918 pandemic passed into pigs in North America, where it still persists and causes winter epidemics of swine influenza (Shope, 1944).

FIGURE 6

The spread of the Asian virus, influenza A/Singapore/57, in the 1957 pandemic

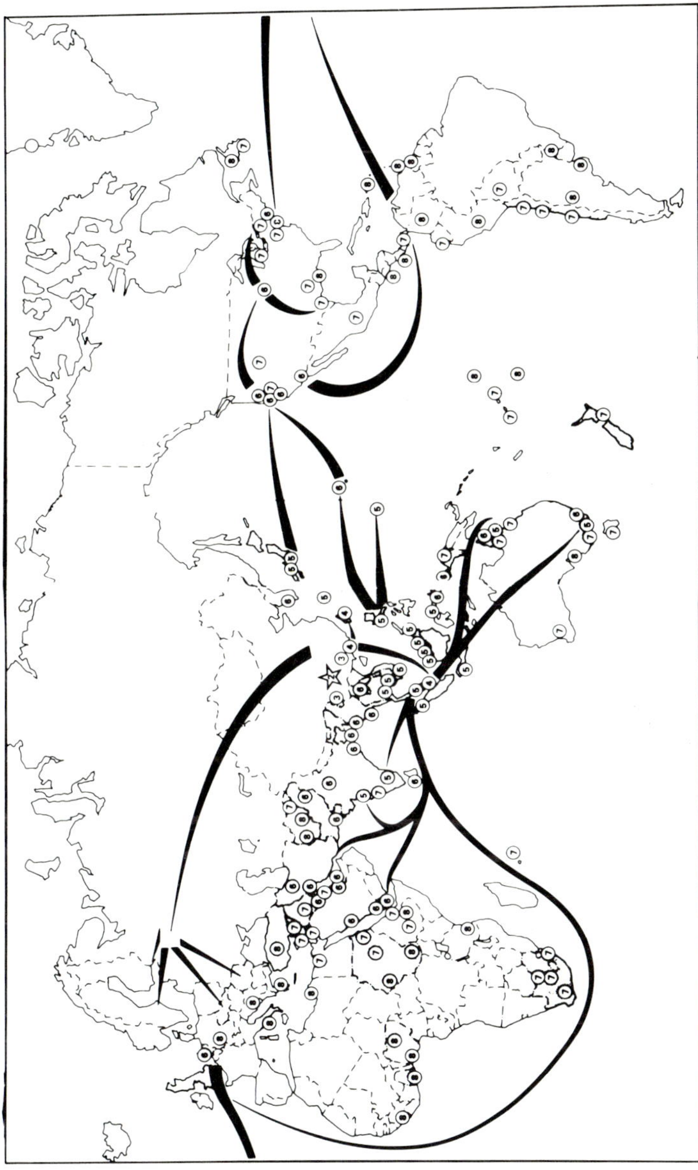

☆ Probable origin of the epidemic.
Numbers in circles refer to the month of the epidemic.
From Stuart-Harris and Schild (1976).

Variability

The incidence of influenza varies from one outbreak to another, and varies with age during any given epidemic. This is well shown by data from Dr Fry's practice in Beckenham (Table 5). The Asian epidemics of 1957 and 1959 both had maximal incidence in children and young adults. In 1959, influenza B may have contributed to the number of affected children. Those in older age groups experienced relatively little influenza in the early epidemics of the Asian virus era. But the antigenically-drifted virus of 1967-68 caused a higher incidence in people over 60 years of age than did the earlier outbreaks, and in England and Wales as a whole mortality was considerable.

The incidence of influenza in semi-isolated communities, such as residential schools or army camps, often differs greatly from the incidence among people living at home. Figure 7 shows an outbreak in a girls' boarding-school near Sheffield, which in 1950 suffered an attack rate of 60%, and two H_1N_1 epidemics in army camps in the midlands, in January 1947. Although the attack rates were only 20%, the explosive build-up of illness was typical of the pattern of influenza in communities where transmission of virus is facilitated by the manner of life. The incidence of influenza in the towns near these camps was only sporadic, and contrasted greatly with the incidence in the camps. As the H_1N_1 virus was then being experienced for the first time, the difference in incidence between civilian and army groups is unlikely to have been immunological.

TABLE 5

Influenza A2 epidemics in a general practice

Virus	*Age group*								*Total*
	0-9	10-19	20-29	30-39	40-49	50-59	60-69	70-79	
1957 A2	27	36	18	13	12	10	9	4	17
1959 A2 + B	25	18	14	14	11	11	8	4	14
1961 A2	1	2	4	4	4	6	3	2	3
1966 B + A2	14	5	6	8	5	6	4	3	7
1967-68 A2	16	6	4	3	5	9	14	10	8
1969 HK	0.2	1.2	1.4	1.1	2.2	3.0	1.6	0.3	1.3

Numbers are attack rates per 100 people at risk, by age group, in successive outbreaks of A2 (Asian, H_2N_2) influenza and one epidemic of A/Hong Kong influenza in 1968-69. From Stuart-Harris and Schild (1976), after Fry (1969 and personal communication).

FIGURE 7

Explosive epidemics of influenza. Influenza A (H_1 N_1) epidemic in army camps, 1947. Influenza B epidemic in a residential school, 1950.

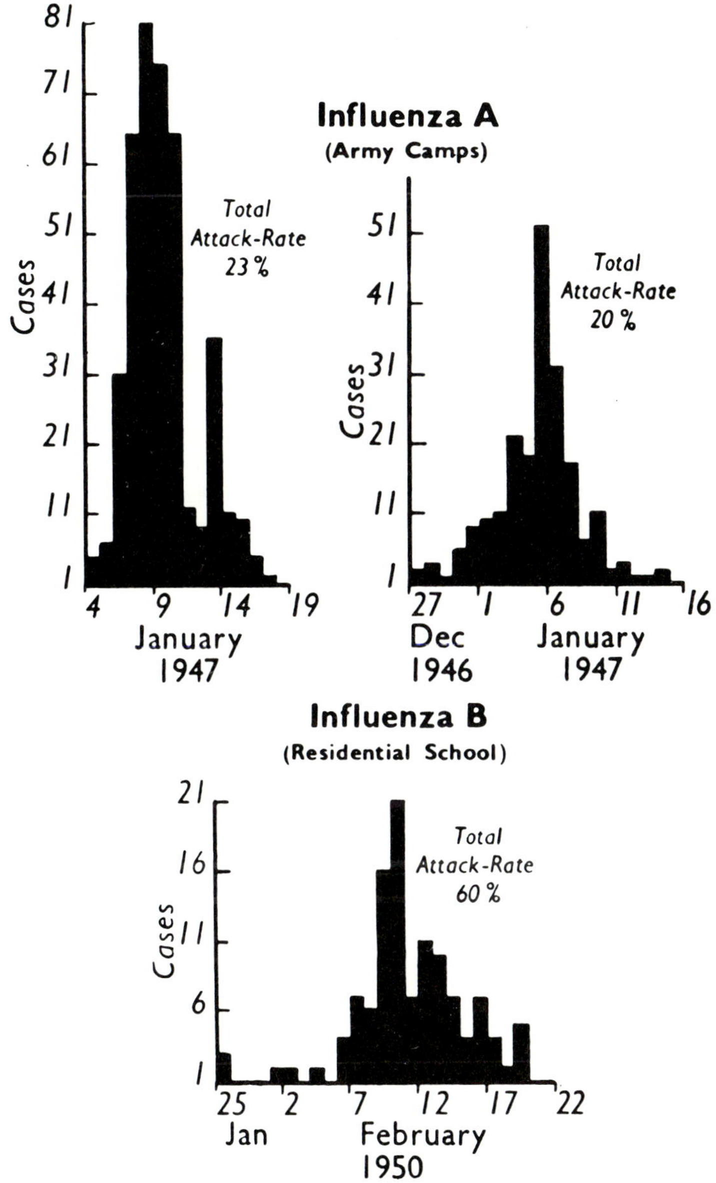

Attack rates are shown in the figure. From Stuart-Harris (1952).

The records of Dr Will Pickles, of Wensleydale, are shown in Figure 8. The Wensleydale valley is studded with small villages, each with a population of a few hundred people. The figure shows the experience of these villages in a single epidemic, in 1937. Some villages escaped with only a handful of cases, but in others there was a sharply-peaked epidemic. Sir Macfarlane Burnet obtained from Pickles the records of influenza in these villages in earlier years (Pickles et al., 1947), and showed that the incidence in previous influenza outbreaks was inversely

FIGURE 8

Pickles' record of influenza outbreaks in villages of Wensleydale, Yorkshire, 1937

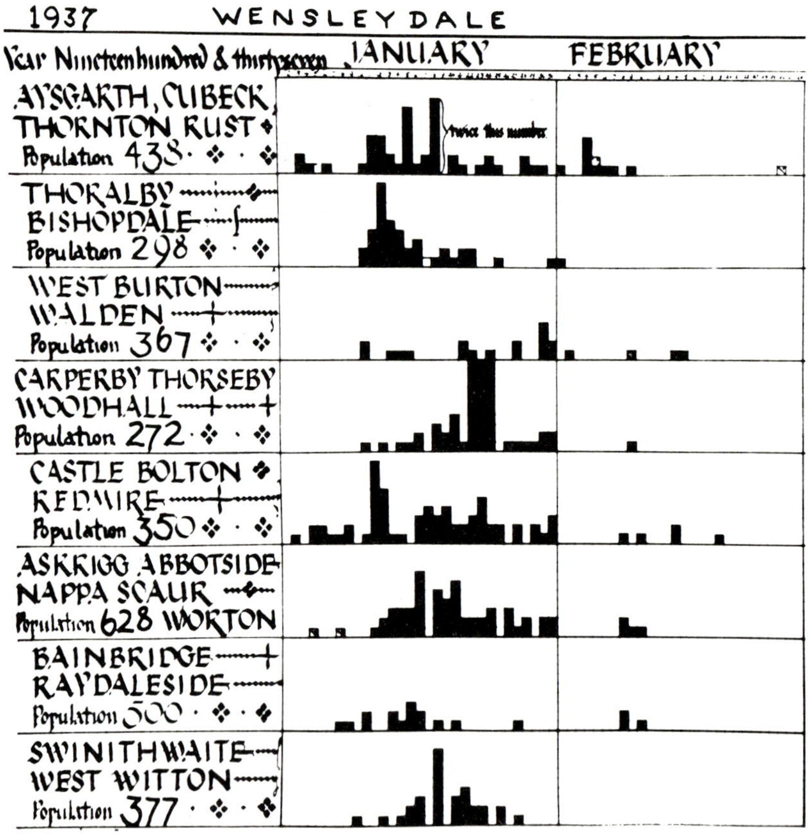

From Stuart-Harris and Schild (1976).

correlated with the incidence in 1937. Clearly, immunological resistance to influenza virus explains some of the variability of outbreaks in different population groups.

References

Cockburn, W. C., Delon, P. J., and Ferreira, W. (1969) *Bull. Wld Hlth Org., 41,* 345.
Francis, T., Jr. (1940) *Science, 92,* 405.
Fry, J. (1969) *J. Roy. Coll. G.P., 17,* 100.
Langmuir, A. D. (1961) *Amer. Rev. resp. Dis., 83,* 2.
Magill, T. P. (1940) *Proc. Soc. Exp. Biol. (N.Y.), 45,* 162.
Masurel, N. C. (1969) *Lancet, i,* 907.
Payne, A. M.-M. (1958) *Proc. Roy. Soc. Med., 51,* 1009.
Pickles, W. N., Burnet, F. M., and McArthur, N. (1947) *J. Hygiene (Camb.), 45,* 469.
Salk, J. E., Menke, W. J., and Francis, T., Jr. (1944) *J. Amer. med. Ass., 124* 93.
Shope, R. E. (1944) *Medicine, 23,* 415.
Stuart-Harris, C. H. (1952) *Influenza,* London: Edward Arnold.
Stuart-Harris, C. H. (1970) *J. inf. Dis., 122,* 108.
Stuart-Harris, C. H. and Schild, G. C. (1976) *Influenza, the viruses and the disease,* London: Edward Arnold.

Epidemiology of influenza: key facts and remaining problems (2)

J. W. G. Smith

ABSTRACT

Epidemiological data on influenza from national returns, although imprecise, have been of great value in conjunction with virological studies in elucidating many of the factors which account for epidemics. This understanding, supplemented by estimates of excess mortality, has been of practical value in deciding vaccination policies. Special studies to provide better epidemiological data are justified if they lead to improvements in forecasting and resource allocation. They are further justified by the expectation that greater epidemiological knowledge will help to identify, and direct the attention of research workers to, the critical factors in the virus, the host, and the environment on which epidemic behavior depends. Modelling should play an important role in identifying these critical factors.

The broad descriptive epidemiology of influenza is well known. The typical picture of a winter outbreak can be plotted graphically using nationally available statistics. Figure 1 shows, for example, the number of diagnoses of influenza reported weekly by "spotter" GPs to the epidemiological unit of the Royal College of General Practitioners (RCGP), paralleled by the number of deaths attributed to influenza on death certificates. These numbers rise and fall in parallel with deaths from all causes. In England, records of new claims for sickness benefit are available on a national basis, and indicate a similar rise and fall in illness in the general adult population. These variations are associated with isolations of influenza virus, reported in England and Wales through the Public Health Laboratory Service (PHLS). Figure 2 shows this descriptive picture plotted year by year, enabling influenza epidemics to be compared.

This sort of information is not difficult to obtain, and comprises the data with which most people working in this field are familiar. Analysis of these simple data, and study of the factors that influence the size and severity of epidemics (characteristics of the virus, the host, and the environment, notably weather and air temperature) have yielded a great deal of understanding without recourse to any modelling whatsoever.

FIGURE 1

Fluctuations in various indicators of influenza activity in the UK, during the winter of 1974-75

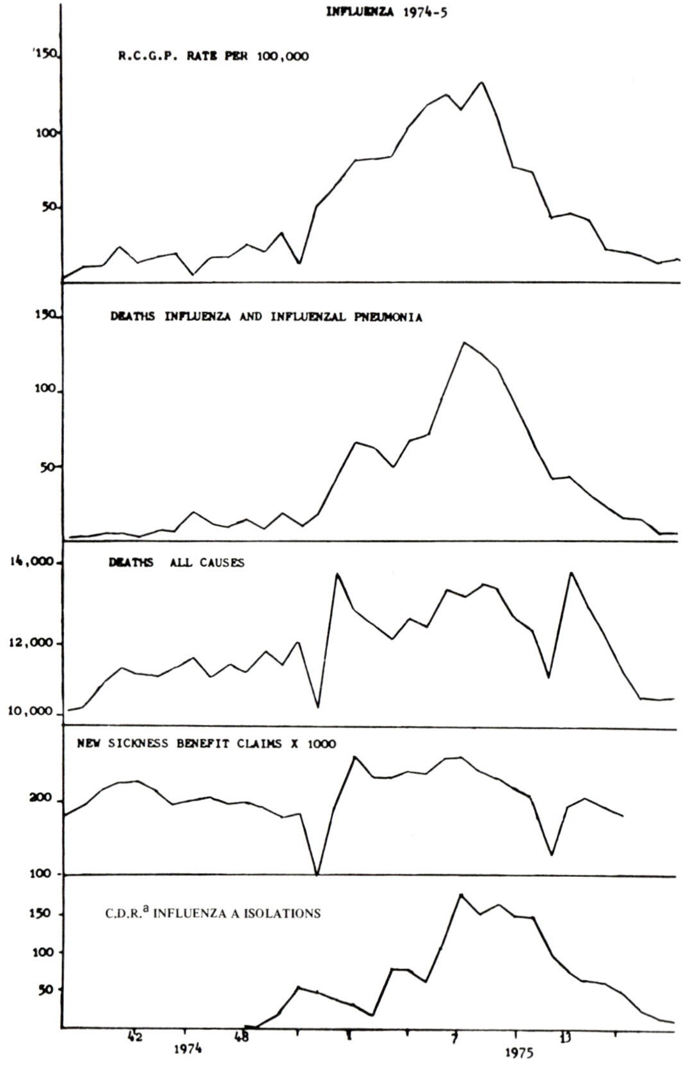

[a] Communicable Disease Report of the Public Health Laboratory Service.

FIGURE 2

Fluctuations in various indicators of influenza activity in the UK, between 1967 and 1975

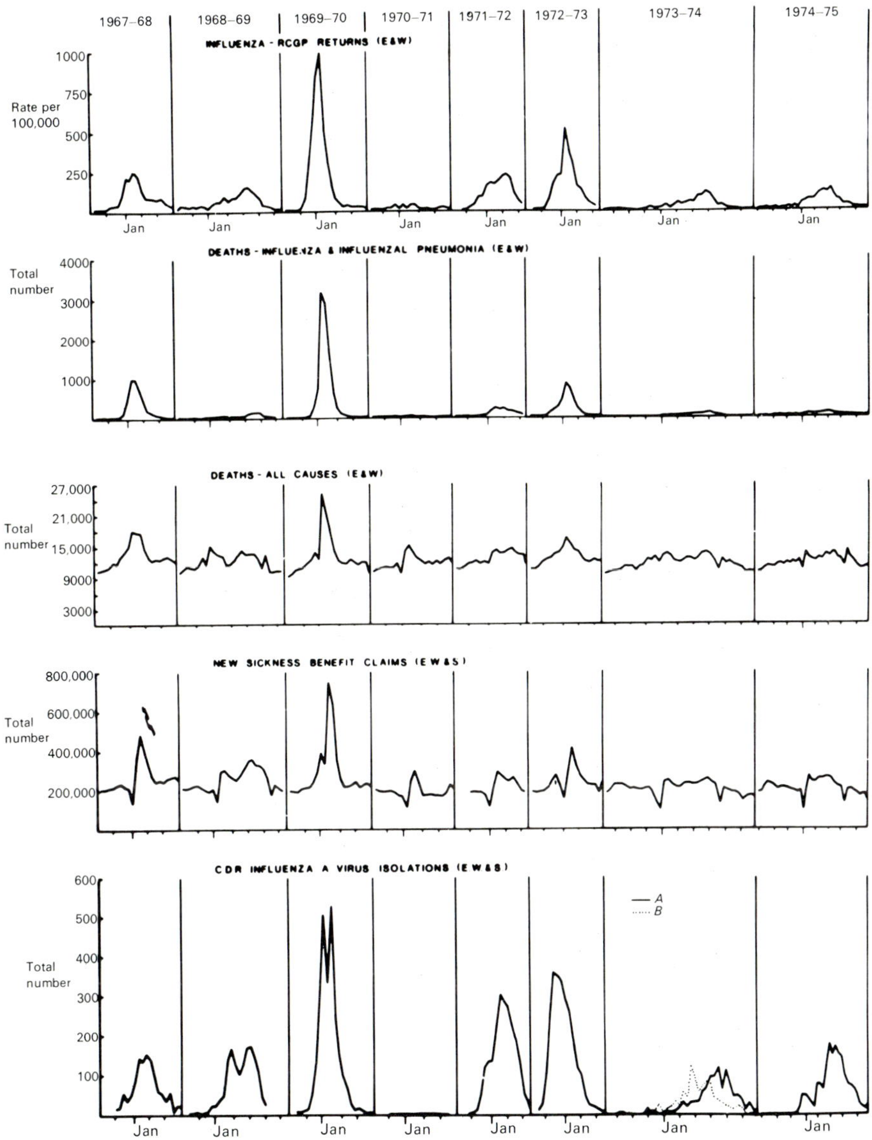

This understanding has influenced current vaccination policies and is used, albeit very inaccurately, to forecast epidemic severity. We know that major factors associated with epidemics are changes in the surface antigens of the virus, weather (influenza usually occurs in the winter), and the immunity level of the human host population, as determined by anti-haemagglutinin antibodies. The simple, nationally-available data have, therefore, provided a rewarding basis for studies of influenza epidemiology.

Figure 3, which may be familiar to you, is Dr Kilbourne's illustration of the introduction of a new virus into a population which has no antibody against it. As a result a pandemic spreads around the world, leading to immunity in some of the population, i.e. those who become infected and recover. The pandemic dies away, possibly owing to environmental factors, before a high level of population immunity has been built up. In the following winter, a smaller epidemic occurs which further increases immunity levels. Subsequent winter epidemics are likely to be set off by small changes in the surface antigens of the pandemic virus (antigenic drift), which enable it to partly overcome the immunity of the population and cause an outbreak. Kilbourne's picture suggests that inter-pandemic outbreaks get smaller as the antibody level in the population builds up, in the way that Sir Charles showed in his Sheffield serological studies. Eventually a new virus breaks through, from causes which we may consider later during the discussion. Now this picture is a reasonable explanation of the observed events, and I would like to ask: Is there any need to go further than just getting this general data? Do we need more detailed epidemiological data?

In my view, the information we have considered so far, i.e. deaths, diagnoses, new sickness benefit claims, and virus isolation reports, is very soft; if you are working on models it is as well to recognize how imprecise these figures are. In England and Wales, it is probably impossible to get a random sample of the population on which to do serological studies; a compromise has to be made, for example using blood donor samples, which by no means accurately represent the general population. Further, the number of virus isolations obtained depends upon the quality of the swabs, the speed with which they are transported to the laboratory, and the standards of the laboratory work. Clinical diagnosis of influenza is also very imprecise. Consequently, the epidemiological picture we have built up must have wide confidence limits, and modellers should be aware of this.

The quality of the epidemiological data could be improved by special studies aimed at improving estimates of the true infection rate and the consequences of infection, i.e. subclinical illness, clinical illness, hospitalization, and death. It would also be possible to study the rate and

FIGURE 3

Decline of severity of influenza epidemics in the post-pandemic period as a function of increased levels of specific (A2) antibody in the exposed population. Subtype-specific immunity leads to the suppression of the A2 variant. Non-A2-like mutants will have survival advantage

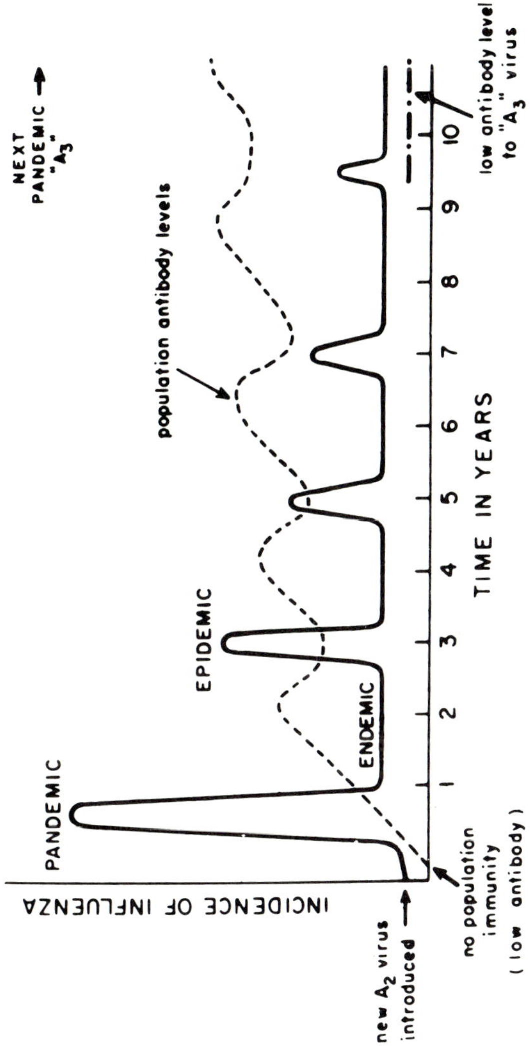

From Kilbourne, E.D. (1973) *J. infect. Dis., 127,* 480.

effects of infection in different groups of the population, broken down by age and social environment, for example to compare dense population centers with villages, or factory workers with schoolchildren. I believe the effort involved in securing such data can be justified on two grounds.

First, if it leads to a better use of preventive and other resources. The information we already have has dictated the use of resources quite significantly. For example, as a result of the knowledge that influenza outbreaks can be very severe in closed communities, and that many deaths may occur in old people's homes, the elderly in institutions are an important target for vaccination. But more detailed epidemiological studies, such as those of Monto and Cavallaro (1971) in Tecumseh, have raised a strong suggestion that vaccination of schoolchildren can affect the impact of influenza on the whole population of a city. If more detailed epidemiological knowledge could lead to a better use of resources, this would be a strong justification for more work on descriptive epidemiology.

Second, and more important, is the possibility that greater epidemiological knowledge can lead to an increased understanding of the causes of epidemiological phenomena. This clearly requires parallel studies of the properties of the virus, the host, and the environment that affect these phenomena. The information we already have points to studies which could be valuable. For example, why are epidemics very severe in closed communities? Is it merely the influence of close contact, or does the virus gain in virulence or transmissibility? A greater knowledge of the epidemiology of influenza could direct research to the critical factors which might explain the epidemiological facts. For example, influenza epidemics are sometimes more severe in one town than another. Collection of data on the antibody distribution in the two populations, before and after the epidemics, and on the social characteristics of the two cities, might suggest that the epidemic differences are due to meteorological differences, the identification of which might be a major advance. This possibility provides a strong justification for the more detailed study of descriptive epidemiology, but it also justifies work on mathematical models. It seems to me that modelling could play an important role in helping to identify the features of the virus, the host, or the environment which could most profitably be studied. For example, a model might indicate whether the amount of virus secreted is more important than the level of susceptibility of the human host, so that progress would then be more likely to come from studies of virus secretion. Modelling could have a significant and productive impact on experimental work on influenza. This impact is likely to be greatest if the data available to modellers are firm and detailed.

I would like to enlarge on this point a little further. The properties of the virus which affect the severity of an epidemic must, I suppose, be related to factors affecting transmission, such as the amount of virus secreted, which Dr Tyrrell will talk about later, and those affecting virulence, which are not yet understood. It is known that the virus has to possess surface antigens to which the susceptible host does not have antibodies, but there must also be other properties which dictate how severely the individual is affected, and understanding these is of practical importance in relation to live vaccines. The environmental qualities affecting transmission must also be important, and the influence of humidity and temperature is clearly open to study. Although we have a good idea of the main determinant of immunity, which is circulating anti-haemagglutinin antibody, there must be other factors in the resistance of the host which we do not know about, perhaps related to cellular immunity or to the amount of secretory antibody present, and these also are open to study. The gaps in knowledge are considerable, and if modelling could enable the more important ones to be identified, then the work of mathematicians would be fully justified.

A more detailed study of what I've called descriptive epidemiology could be a formidable undertaking, owing to the imprecision of the diagnosis of influenza and of the identification of the consequences of infection. One method of study, used by the PHLS, involved a group of general practitioners whose practices were scattered over the country. They reported to a central laboratory the age and sex structure of their practice population (Figure 4), this being possible in the UK because, under the national health service, patients register with their doctors. The GPs then reported weekly the number of first consultations for acute respiratory illness, broken down by sex and age (Figure 5). They also took swabs from a proportion of these patients every week. The swabs were then sent for virus culture by collaborating laboratories, where the best available methods for influenza viruses were used.

The sort of data this yielded is illustrated in Table 1. The acute respiratory consultation rate can be calculated each week. The number of swabs examined is recorded. In the winter of 1973-74, for example, 360 swabs were examined in the 0-4 year age group, of which 2.2% yielded influenza A and 2.8% influenza B. This virus isolation rate was used to determine the "virologically estimated attack rate", which was about 3 % for the whole of that outbreak and could be regarded as a fairly close approximation to the number of virologically positive cases of influenza. The week-by-week picture in 1974-75 is illustrated graphically in Figure 6.

But even this type of information, which requires much effort to gain, is imprecise. It refers only to those people who actually go to their doctor with an illness, and disregards the many people who have a mild

FIGURE 4

Form for reporting age and sex structure of practice population

PHLS INFLUENZA SURVEILLANCE Form IS E3

ENTRY DATA FOR GENERAL PRACTICE
PARTICIPATING IN SCHEME

NAME OF DOCTORS ____________________

Location ____________________

Main Surgery ____________________

Tel. No. ____________

Person supplying information: ____________________

AGE/SEX STRUCTURE OF PRACTICE AS AT __________ 197__		
Age Group (Years)	Males	Females
Under 5		
5 - 14		
15 - 24		
25 - 44		
45 - 64		
65 & over		
Not known		
Total		

Official number of patients as per Executive Council list on June 30th 1973:-

Total patients

Number 65 years and over ________

FIGURE 5

Form for weekly reporting of numbers of first consultations for acute respiratory illness, by age and sex

PHLS — Form IS 3

INFLUENZA SURVEILLANCE

FIRST CONSULTATIONS OF PATIENTS SUFFERING WITH ACUTE RESPIRATORY ILLNESS

Practice: ______________ Week ended Friday ______________ 197

	AGE GROUP OF PATIENTS SEEN (YEARS)							
	Under 5	5 - 14	15 - 24	25 - 44	45 - 64	65 & over	Not known	Total
MALES								
FEMALES								
Total								

TABLE 1

Age distribution of total cases of acute respiratory illness seen from week 45 (1973) to 18 (1974), together with results of virus culture for influenza A and B

	Age group					
	0-4	*5-14*	*15-24*	*25-44*	*45-64*	*65 +*
Acute respiratory consultation rate per 100,000 in surveillance practices	62,400	27,100	16,200	12,600	11,100	11,100
Number of swabs examined	360	698	461	812	367	89
% swabs +ve influenza A	2.2	2.2	3.0	4.6	4.4	3.4
Virologically estimated influenza A rate per 100,000	1,370	600	490	580	490	380
% swabs +ve influenza B	2.8	8.6	3.5	3.3	3.8	4.5
Virologically estimated influenza B rate per 100,000	1,750	2,330	570	420	420	500
Virologically estimated influenza A and B rate per 100,000	3,120	2,930	1,060	1,000	910	880

attack of influenza and do not bother their doctor. The results also depend on the reliability of virus isolation, and this is an uncertain element which could vary between epidemics and, possibly, between the beginning and end of an epidemic. It is not impossible that more virus is secreted by patients attacked at the height of an epidemic than at the end, and this would affect the isolation of virus from swabs.

Virus isolation from swabs can be supplemented by serological diagnosis, but this is difficult in a large population. A five-year study was set up by the RCGP, using volunteer families from whom blood samples were taken before and after each winter and who were intensively studied virologically in the event of illness. Unfortunately, during the five years of the study there was no large outbreak. It is a major task to mount and successfully maintain detailed population studies, and the work can largely be wasted if influenza outbreaks do not occur. Perhaps, by the end

FIGURE 6

Weekly fluctuations in acute respiratory illness rate, percentage of swabs positive for influenza virus, and virologically estimated influenza rate, in 1974-75

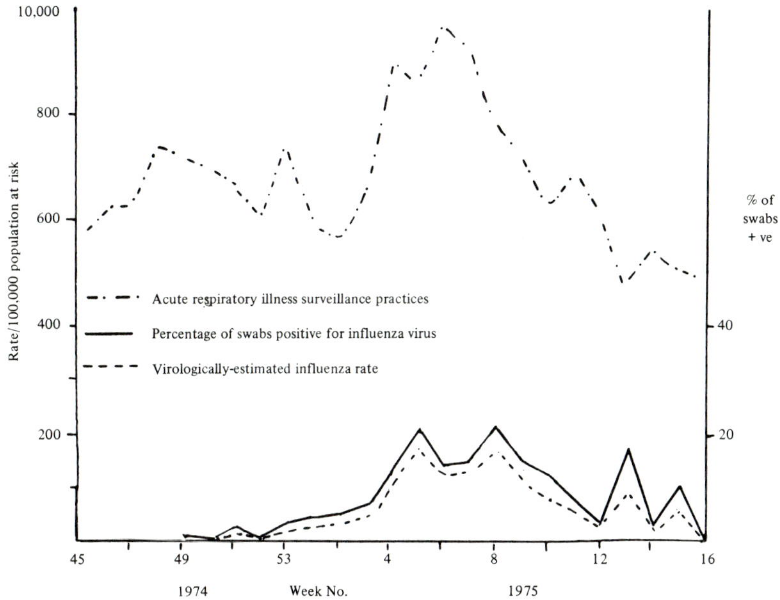

of this meeting, we shall be able to forecast epidemics accurately so that we could mount such studies at the right time!

The PHLS studies, like the studies in Tecumseh and elsewhere, have shown repeatedly that the attack rate is often highest in young children (Figure 7). This is usually explained by the fact that young children tend to cough over each other, are in close contact, and are usually serologically susceptible once they have lost maternal antibody. But it is also possible that they secrete virus more readily, and that the high attack rates seen in young children are in part an artifact due to easier virus isolations.

One of the points which has come out of the influenza surveillance work of the PHLS is that the RCGP diagnoses, based on "spotter" practices, give a surprisingly accurate picture of the amount of clinical influenza. The clinical diagnosis of influenza is difficult, being more accurate in bigger epidemics and less accurate in small outbreaks, in which influenza merges with the background of acute respiratory infection due to

FIGURE 7

Virologically estimated incidence of clinical influenza by age group, in England and Wales

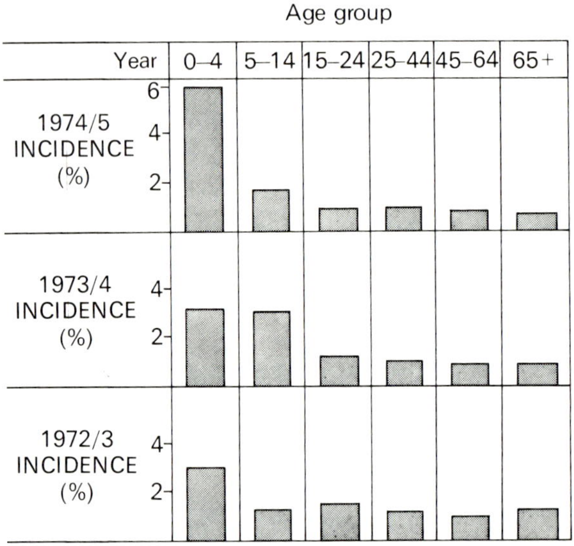

From Public Health Laboratory Service Standing Committee on Influenza (1977) *J. Hygiene (Camb.), 78,* 223.

other causes. But despite this difficulty, the clinical diagnoses made by the "spotter" doctors seem to give a reliable picture of outbreaks.

Study of deaths from influenza has been of value. Table 2 shows the number of deaths attributed to influenza and influenzal pneumonia on death certificates, in England and Wales. But we know that this is a very imprecise measure, as the early studies on excess mortality by

TABLE 2

Deaths attributed to influenza and influenzal pneumonia on death certificates, in England and Wales

Number of deaths due to influenza and influenzal pneumonia in the epidemiological year							
1967-68	*1968-69*	*1969-70*	*1970-71*	*1971-72*	*1972-73*	*1973-74*	*1974-75*[a]
4,710	1,428	10,274	471	1,882	3,904	1,140	1,366

William Farr (1847) in London showed. Studies of excess mortality, using estimates based on regression analysis, have been made in England and Wales. In 1974-75, for example, whilst deaths attributed to influenza on death certificates numbered about 1,400, excess mortality was about 29,000 (Table 3). In the UK, we are also able to study excess new claims for sickness benefit as an estimate of morbidity in working-age adults. But this is a very rough estimate, because people's motives for claiming sickness benefit are not always due to influenza; they may take advantage of an epidemic to have a week off work.

TABLE 3

Influenza in successive winters from 1968 to 1975

	1968-69	*1969-70*	*1970-71*	*1971-72*	*1972-73*	*1973-74*	*1974-75*[a]
Influenza cases/100,000 from RCGP returns, weeks 38-24 (E, W, and S)	1,802	4,297	594	2,016	2,641	1,220	1,630
Deaths attributed to influenza and influenzal pneumonia reported to Registrar General, weeks 38-24 (E and W)	1,387	10,209	433	1,877	3,885	1,132	1,335
Excess mortality from all causes, weeks 38-24 (E and W)	20,000	27,635	0	11,037	19,372	18,000	29,480
Excess new sickness benefit claims, weeks 38-24, in millions (E, W, and S)	1.8	2.2	0	0	1.0	0.6	0.6

E and W = England and Wales. E, W, and S = England, Wales, and Scotland.

[a] 1974-75 figures refer to weeks 38-21.

One point which emerges clearly from studies of excess mortality is the high proportion of deaths in old people during influenza epidemics. In 1971-72, for example, there were 16,000 excess deaths at all ages, of which 15,500 were in the elderly (Table 4). This tendency, as you know, has been used in justifying the US policy of advocating influenza vaccine for everybody over the age of 65 years. More recent estimates of excess mortality are available for England and Wales (Table 5), but there were only small epidemics in recent years and these estimates may be very inaccurate. Further study of excess mortality is justified, in practical terms, if it leads to the better identification of high-risk groups, such as diabetics, who could become target groups for vaccination.

TABLE 4

Mortality in excess of that in non-influenza winters, in England and Wales, for people aged 65 years and over and for all ages

	Excess mortality, 1 September–31 May	
	65 years and over	*All ages*
Excess mortality calculated by comparison with influenza-free winter of 1966-67		
1964-65	3,866	9,038
1965-66	27,446	35,019
1966-67	0	0
1967-68	43,838	48,028
Excess mortality calculated by comparison with influenza-free winter of 1970-71		
1968-69	3,037	8,796
1969-70	18,836	26,319
1970-71	0	0
1971-72	15,552	16,097

TABLE 5

Estimates of excess deaths and excess new sickness benefit claims attributable to influenza, in England and Wales (weeks 41-20)

Winter	*Excess total deaths from all causes*	*Excess deaths from respiratory causes*	*Excess deaths in 65 + age group, from all causes*	*Excess new claims for sickness benefit (× 1,000)*
1975-76	22,250	17,210	19,590	908
1976-77	4,060	5,790	[a]	322
1977-78	5,910	6,080	[a]	364
1978-79	5,430	5,500	[a]	237
Approximate standard error of estimates	5,000	2,500	4,300	225

[a]Data not available.
From Tillett, H. E., Smith, J. W. G., and Clifford, R. E. (1980) *Lancet*, *i*, 793.

In summary, the epidemiological data we derive from nationally-available returns is imprecise. It has, nevertheless, been of great value in conjunction with studies of the virus, the host, and the environment in elucidating many of the factors which account for epidemics of influenza.

It has already proved its practical value in influencing vaccination policies, especially when supplemented by estimates of excess mortality. More detailed and precise epidemiological data can be obtained by special studies which involve collaboration between laboratories and GPs, and which are time-consuming. Such work is of value for its own sake, but is further justified if it leads to improvement in forecasting, and in deciding where best to allocate resources, which in practice mainly means vaccine. Its main justification, however, is that greater epidemiological knowledge may lead to identification of the critical factors responsible for the behavior of the virus in the population, and thereby stimulate research into these factors. In this process, modelling should have an important role to play in identifying those critical features of the virus, the host, or the environment in which laboratory or field studies should prove most rewarding.

References

Farr, W. (1847) *Tenth annual report of the Registrar General*, London: HMSO.

Monto, A.S., and Cavallaro, J.J. (1971) *Amer. J. Epid.*, *94*, 280.

Session I: Discussion of presentations by Stuart-Harris and J. Smith

Rapporteur: J. Smith

Tyrell said that the factors leading to the decline of outbreaks were not well understood, but that seasonal conditions probably played an important part. Epidemics often decline at a time when there are still many susceptibles in the population.

Stuart-Harris agreed that the factors involved in the cessation of epidemics needed study, and were possibly as important as those leading to their upsurge.

Spicer asked whether there was doubt about the precision of estimates of the incidence of infection, based upon serological diagnoses.

Stuart-Harris replied that the evidence indicated that roughly 50% of influenza infections were sub-clinical. While infections might occur that are not detected by conventional serological tests, they are probably unimportant. The significance of serological data as an indicator of attack rates is supported by the evidence of resistance in people with antibodies. If infection occurs without antibody formation, it is not apparently accompanied by the development of immunity.

Tyrrell pointed out that the two presentations mainly concerned UK experience, and asked for information on influenza surveillance in other countries.

Choi described the CDC (Centers for Disease Control) national surveillance program based on reported deaths from influenza, from pneumonia, and from all causes in 121 cities in different parts of the USA. The cities include 26% of the country's population, and account for about one-third of the total deaths.

There is no US scheme comparable to that of the RCGP (Royal College of General Practitioners) in the UK. A commercial firm, IMS, operates a survey for marketing purposes. It involves 15,000 doctors scattered throughout the USA, who each report their practice records for two days every quarter in such a way that a report is made for each day of the year. However, each daily report concerns a very small sample of the US population.

This survey probably gives a reasonable *quarterly* estimate of the number of influenza diagnoses made. The data collected include the causes of consultations and prescribing information.

Choi commented that, despite the "softness" of certain data such as deaths as an index of influenza activity, the data are consistently available and can be used to compare seasons and to indicate trends.

Spicer pointed out that the Russian surveillance data are based on the daily notification of clinical diagnoses of acute respiratory disease, by doctors working in polyclinics.

Choi, Stuart-Harris, and others referred to an additional US source of data, the "health interview study", based on interviews by health workers. The accuracy of the clinical diagnoses made is probably much lower than that made by doctors, especially those who volunteered to report to the RCGP scheme in the UK.

Elveback referred to the value of the Tecumseh study and the Seattle virus watch, in which small numbers of volunteer families were kept under careful surveillance, supplemented by clinical and virological investigations. In the Seattle study, a nurse called on each family weekly and a "sentinel" provided a throat swab for virus culture. If an illness occurred in any family member, all the family provided a swab. Serum samples were collected six-monthly. Dr Longini has analyzed the Seattle serological family data on H_1N_1, H_3N_2, and influenza B viruses.

Choi said that influenza findings from the Seattle study were currently being analyzed.

Fine drew the discussion back to the natural history of the disease, and raised two questions. Firstly, why did influenza suddenly appear in 1890, after an interval of about 40 years? Could this have been a reporting artifact?

Stuart-Harris thought this was unlikely, in view of the large increase in deaths in 1890 in the absence of any change in the reporting methods in the UK at that time.

Fine's second point concerned the apparently novel circumstance of the simultaneous circulation of H_1N_1 and H_3N_2 viruses in the last five years. Previously it was accepted that only one antigenic subtype circulated at any one time. Could this change signal a new development in influenza epidemiology, or were the earlier views incorrect?

Stuart-Harris commented that current influenza epidemiology, with different subtypes and lesser antigenic variants all circulating in the population at the same time, was ill understood. He recalled that Isaacs isolated an H_1N_1 virus on one occasion in about 1958, from a solider, but there was no other evidence that an epidemiological picture like the present one had been observed previously.

Tyrrell said that, in his view, the situation revealed by recent virological studies accorded better with biological expectations, based on the behavior of other viruses, than did the rapid and apparently complete disappearance of an influenza subtype from the world. This view was supported by J. Smith.

Tyrrell referred to the importance of anti-haemagglutinin antibody as proved by current experience with H_1 viruses, which are confined to age groups too young to have experienced H_1 viruses previously.

Stuart-Harris knew of only one example of a breakthrough of immunity derived from past H_1 experience, an outbreak of H_1N_1 influenza in a geriatric group, in 1979.

J. Smith observed that the resistance of older people to H_1 strains also demonstrated the long duration of immunity provided by natural influenza infection.

Stuart-Harris mentioned that H_1N_1 influenza in young people is fairly mild clinically. Also, the present virus strains are more sensitive to the temperature of incubation when grown in tissue culture, than are other wild strains of influenza virus.

Bachmayer pointed out that clinical diagnoses, even when based on the reports of selected doctors, remain an imprecise source for estimates of the influenza attack rate.

Abstract of discussion

1. The factors leading to the decline of epidemics are ill understood. They may be as interesting and important as those leading to the onset of epidemics.

2. About 50% of infections are sub-clinical. Serological surveys provide a fairly reliable index of the overall attack rate.

3. Serum anti-haemagglutinin antibody provides a fairly good index of immunity to attack.

4. Although national data concerning the effects of influenza are crude, they provide a valuable basis for modelling.

5. More precise and more detailed data require special studies, such as those exemplified by the Seattle virus watch.

6. The recent observation of more than one subtype of virus circulating simultaneously may be a new phenomenon which is ill understood. Biologically, however, such behavior is more to be expected than the complete disappearance of a subtype.

Session II

Models of the temporal spread of epidemics

Bailey

Spicer

L. Smith

Choi

Models of the temporal spread of epidemics (1)

N. T. J. Bailey

ABSTRACT

Basically, models can be envisaged in terms of boxes labelled 'susceptibles', 'infectives', 'immunes', etc., with individuals moving at certain rates from box to box. At this stage, agreement must be reached between epidemiologists and their mathematical advisors. Once the flow-rates are specified, the behavior of the system can be calculated in terms of mathematics, possibly computer-assisted. Results can later be interpreted back into epidemiological or public health terms. A special characteristic of infectious disease modelling, leading to many technical difficulties, is the typical 'mass-action' phenomenon.

It is useful to distinguish 'functional' models, in which purely statistical methods must be used for the broad interpretation of highly aggregated data, from disaggregated, 'structural' micro-modelling, which handles the underlying mechanisms of the spread of infection.

The satisfactory solution of many practical problems depends on answers to theoretical questions. However, much more detailed biomathematical work is required on individual diseases, and influenza in particular, in order to permit adequate statistical estimation, hypothesis testing, and model validation. Increased emphasis must also be given to practical questions of disease control, such as optimal choice of alternative strategies and resource allocation.

1. General remarks

For a detailed review of the broad implications of the application of mathematical models to the dynamics of the spread of infectious diseases in general, and influenza in particular, we must of course refer to Paul Fine's excellent background paper. In the present introduction, intended to initiate and stimulate discussion, I shall therefore only touch on a restricted set of special features that it may be useful to bear in mind. There is, in fact, a huge literature on the specifically mathematical theory of infectious diseases (see Bailey, 1975), now totalling at least 700 references. Moreover, this total has been increasing in recent years at a rate that is faster than exponential. The amount of work concerned directly with influenza modelling is naturally much more limited, and currently runs to some 25-30 references (this total is of course much larger if we include a wide variety of statistical analyses).

2. Types of models

The various types of possible modelling that have been described appear at first sight to be highly diverse, and Fine (*loc. cit.*) gives a partial classification of some of the alternatives available. Actually, many of these are not fundamentally different, but simply indicate a variety of special features that might or might not be included. For a more detailed discussion of modelling see Bailey (1977), Chapter 5. In practice, it is useful first to distinguish two major phases, as follows.

First, often as a result of prolonged discussion between epidemiologists and their mathematical/statistical advisors, some kind of consensus is arrived at in which a qualitative picture emerges, consisting largely of a set of boxes or compartments representing epidemiological states. Thus we may have susceptibles, infectious individuals, people who have recovered and are immune, carriers, etc. Any given individual may be thought of as moving at some rate to be defined from one box to another. So far, this picture, or model, is largely qualitative, and is based on direct perceptions and intuitions.

At this stage we have what is essentially a flow-chart, and there should be little difficulty in pursuing general arguments and discussions in terms of ordinary commonsense approaches using everyday language plus a minimum number of standard epidemiological concepts.

Next, questions must be faced as to the rates at which individuals move from box to box. These may be related to some specific interactions, like that between susceptibles and infectious persons leading to new infections, or they may be related to the time spent in any one box, like the average rate of conversion from 'latent' to 'infectious' being equal to the reciprocal of the latent period. As soon as all the rates are specified, either numerically or algebraically, we have the essential ingredients of a quantitative model.

We still have something that can be thought about, or interpreted, in epidemiological terms, but at the same time the temporal behavior of the whole process can be described in quantitative mathematical language, using differential equations if the time variable is continuous, or difference equations if it is discrete.

From then on, the detailed logical implications of the assumptions can be derived by strict mathematical argument. We may use exact methods, or approximations when these are not available, and are quite likely to supplement these with various kinds of computer-assisted calculations. An important aspect of all this technical work is that it will normally be possible to interpret the mathematical results in terms of the epidemiological concepts embodied in the initial flow-chart. This means that the results are not only accessible to epidemiological discussion, but that they can be compared in suitable circumstances with relevant data, thus providing methods of testing and validating the model in question.

One special aspect of the majority of infectious disease models that needs mentioning is that they exemplify a typical 'mass-action' activity, as found for example in chemical kinetics. In the present case it is commonly assumed that the rate at which new infections occur is equal to the product of the infection rate, the number of susceptibles, and the number of infectives. The product of the last two variable quantities constitutes a major non-linearity in the process, and this leads to all kinds of technical complications.

All of the above principles can be greatly extended and developed, but it is easy to see how the study of temporal spread arises quite naturally. The problem of dealing with spatial aspects will be taken up explicitly in Session VI.

3. Structural versus functional approaches

Two substantially different, though sometimes interacting, approaches that arise quite naturally are the following. The first arises when we study macro-phenomena, such as the total number of cases of disease arising over a certain geographic area and aggregated over a convenient time-interval. Thus we might have the weekly notifications of influenza for a large town, or even a whole country. Little can be said about the detailed aspects of the transmission of disease from one person to another. But we do have an overall, statistical, time-series picture of the temporal flow of events. We may be able, for instance, to observe broad epidemic outbreaks or quasi-regular oscillations in endemic level. Statistical analysis of these patterns may lead to some understanding of the observed data, and this in turn may allow useful predictions to be made, at least in an approximate way.

The models arising from such an approach are often called 'functional', since they aim at describing observed functional patterns more or less directly.

An alternative approach tries to handle underlying mechanisms, seen as the fundamental source of mere surface phenomena. This attempt to penetrate the 'black box' can be exceedingly powerful, since a knowledge of underlying mechanisms, e.g. the law of mass action just referred to, often serves to unify very diverse surface phenomena. It frequently happens in infectious disease epidemiology that enough is known, at least in qualitative terms, of the underlying physiological, biological, or demographic processes for quite acceptable models of structural mechanisms to be developed.

This approach to disaggregated micro-modelling is often called 'structural', because it tries to elucidate the underlying structures and mechanisms.

The distinction between these two approaches is an important one in practice. Quite different types of models are liable to arise, but we should be able to understand how they are related, and which one is appropriate to available data possibly involving both temporally and spatially distributed processes.

The contrast between functional and structural models is relatively straightforward in infectious disease epidemiology, and does not really raise any controversial issues. The same can be said for many other dynamic processes in biology, whereas in applications to anthropology, linguistics, literature, psychology, etc. opposing theories are often hotly debated.

4. General theory and specific applications

A highly prominent aspect of the mathematical literature dealing with infectious diseases is that most of it, perhaps 80%, appears to be almost entirely mathematics, while no more than 20% bears any reference to actual diseases and real data about them.

This is a serious matter, since although some of the mathematical theory is of practical importance, much is mere esoterica. There are in fact many practical problems whose satisfactory solution depends on answers to theoretical questions. So if the latter are solved, real-life issues are affected.

To begin with, we need more insight into the quantitative dynamics of the spread of infectious diseases. This is equally true of macro-epidemics (e.g. the Russian model of influenza spread) and of micro-epidemics involving statistical distributions of different patterns of intra-household spread (e.g. the well-known chain-binomial applications in measles). Many questions arise about qualitatively different kinds of phenomena, such as epidemic or endemic thresholds, probability of fade-out, effect of spatial factors, existence of epidemic waves, sensitivity of results to uncertainty in assumptions about parametric values, etc.

Such questions are often best investigated to begin with through theoretical studies. But the latter must contain a sufficient number of real-life features for qualitative implications to be worked out for actual diseases. There is, therefore, quite a large body of general theory that is of practical importance. A case in point is the question of whether standard 'control theory' can be used to aid practical decision-making. In principle the answer is 'yes', but in practice real-life resource-allocation problems are liable to be too complex for the theory to apply. Nevertheless, theoretical investigations, suitably interpreted, may clarify the issues at stake and suggest approaches that might otherwise be missed.

At the same time, it must be admitted that general theory has far outstripped specific applications. What we need, therefore, is more detailed biomathematical studies of individual diseases. A lot of work has already been done on malaria and measles, for example. In the context of the present meeting it seems highly likely that a connected series of investigations into influenza will be seen to be required.

It is only in studying specific diseases, on which we have suitable data, that general theories and hypotheses can really be tested. Relevant parameters must be estimated, standard errors calculated, chi-squared goodness-of-fit tests carried out to test hypotheses, future predictions made to check verifiability, etc. Model validation can, in short, be achieved only for specific diseases. Moreover, substantive work on disease control, optimal choice of alternative strategies, resource allocation problems, etc. cannot be given concrete interpretations except in relation to concrete examples of individual disease.

References

Bailey, N.T.J. (1975) *The mathematical theory of infectious diseases,* London: Griffin.
Bailey, N.T.J. (1977) *Mathematics, statistics, and systems for health,* Chichester: Wiley.

Models of the temporal spread of epidemics (2)

C. C. Spicer

ABSTRACT

A comprehensive mathematical model of the behavior of influenza epidemics has been developed in the USSR. It covers not merely the form of the epidemic in single cities, but also the spread of disease between cities, taking into account the volume of traffic between them. This latter factor makes it possible to forecast the spread of influenza across the USSR. A remarkable fact is that the parameters describing the epidemic curve in the first city infected are applicable, without modification, to subsequently infected cities. These parameters are only stable within an epidemic year, and differ from year to year. Using this model, the Russians have been able to forecast with reasonable accuracy the intensity of the epidemic in individual cities and the timing of the peak. They have used this information as a basis for administrative action.

A slight modification of the basic model, excluding inter-city spread, has been applied, retrospectively, to data for deaths from influenza and influenzal pneumonia in England and Wales and in Greater London. This has given a reasonable fit to the observed deaths, but its validity as a model of the actual epidemic process is uncertain.

For some years, mathematical methods have been used in the USSR for forecasting the course of influenza epidemics. The methods have been described in a recent book (in Russian) by Baroyan et al. (1977), which gives details of the mathematical model and the accuracy with which it fits the data. A brief report in English has been published by Baroyan et al. (1971), and an account is also given by Bailey (1975).

The Russian system covers two processes: the spread of influenza epidemics between cities, and the behavior of the epidemic wave in individual cities. These are incorporated into a large set of differential equations, which include the rates of migration between cities. The most striking feature of the model is that the main parameter describing the spread of the epidemic within a city is roughly the same for all the main cities of the USSR during the same epidemic year. This parameter is composite, and is the product of the initial number of susceptibles at the start of the epidemic and a factor which depends on the transmissibility and infectivity of the virus.

The Russian model, which closely resembles that put forward by Kermack and McKendrick (1927), is based on the assumption that the rate of progress of the epidemic is proportional to the product of the numbers of susceptible persons and infective cases. This simple assumption has been shown repeatedly in the past to hold remarkably well in practice, for example for measles and the common cold. Further information can be found in Bailey (1975).

The type of calculation used in practice is illustrated in Figure 1. It can be seen that the number of infectious persons in the population at a given moment is equal to the number of those infected in each previous time-interval multiplied by the probability that they survive as infectious cases until that moment. The infectivity of the cases, measured by λ, is taken to be constant at all stages of the disease.

The product:

$$\lambda \cdot S \cdot C$$

(where S and C are the numbers of susceptibles and infectives, respectively) is the number of new cases appearing at a given moment, and this is subtracted from the existing number of susceptibles.

Although the underlying process is strictly a continuous one, in practice it is always necessary to work in finite units, such as a day or a week. In these circumstances, the equation of the epidemic (using the notation of Figure 1) can be written in the form:

$$C_{t+1} = \lambda S_t \sum_{T=0}^{t} C_{t-T}\psi_t$$

$$S_{t+1} = S_t - C_{t+1}$$

FIGURE 1

Diagram illustrating the epidemic model used in this paper

t	*Number still infectious at each stage of illness*	*Susceptible individuals (S)*	*New cases (C)*
0	C_0	S_0	
1	$C_1 \quad C_0\psi_0$	$S_0 - C = S_1$	$C_1 = \lambda S_0 C_0 \psi_0$
2	$C_2 \quad C_1\psi_0 \quad C_0\psi_1$	$S_0 - C_0 - C_1 = S_2$	$C_2 = \lambda S_1 (C_1\psi_0 + C_0\psi_1)$
3	$C_3 \quad C_2\psi_0 \quad C_1\psi_1 \quad C_0\psi_2$	$S_0 - C_0 - C_1 - C_2 = S_3$	$C_3 = \lambda S_2 (C_2\psi_0 + C_1\psi_1 + C_0\psi_2)$

S_t: susceptible individuals at time t
C_t: new cases at time t
ψ_j: proportion of cases still infectious j intervals after being infected
λ : transmissibility parameter

When applying these equations, it is necessary to have estimates of S_0 and C_0 (the initial numbers of susceptibles and infectives, respectively) and also of λ. The value of S_0 is implicit in all the stages of calculating the model and is closely linked to λ, since the course of the epidemic is determined by the product λS_0 and not by the individual values of λ and S_0. For example, an epidemic starting with one million susceptibles and $\lambda = 10^{-6}$ will have the same course as one with 100 susceptibles and $\lambda = 10^{-2}$, provided the initial number of infectives, C_0, is the same.

The function ψ_t, describing the rate at which infectious cases disappear, must be derived from epidemiological studies. Baroyan et al. (1977) have specified the values they used. These imply that no patient is infectious for more than six days.

The full Russian model, which includes the spread between cities, would probably not be applicable to western Europe even if the migration rates between the main cities were known. However, it seemed possible that the equations used for individual cities might be applicable to England and Wales, where mixing of the population is relatively rapid and extensive. A difficulty here is that the only available data relate to deaths from influenza and influenzal pneumonia. By making the simple assumption that the total influenza death rate is constant during an epidemic, and using published figures for the distribution of times of death after infection (Stuart-Harris et al., 1950), it is possible to test the applicability of the model to experience in England and Wales, and also to data for Greater London.

Details of this are given in Spicer (1979). The adequacy with which the model fits the data can be judged from Figure 2. It is clear, when fitted retrospectively, that the general course of the epidemics is quite well described. Certainly, the accuracy of fit is of about the same order as that described by Baroyan et al. for the USSR; their main criteria were that the height of the epidemic peak should be predicted to within ± 30%, and the time of the peak to within ± 5 days.

The values of the composite parameter λS_0 are given in the table.

From a practical point of view, the importance of these results depends upon the interpretability of the parameters in terms of objectively measurable quantities. It is unlikely that the course of an epidemic could be accurately predicted from the first two or three weeks' experience, as the number of cases is relatively small and erratic (i.e. strongly affected by random errors), and the accuracy of diagnosis is low. On the other hand, if information were available on the initial number of susceptibles (S_0) and the infectivity parameter (λ), forecasting might be more reliable. In my opinion, the most fruitful aspect of the model is the light it might throw on the natural history of epidemic influenza. If, in a series of epidemics in communities,

FIGURE 2

Weekly deaths from influenza and influenzal pneumonia in (a) England and Wales and (b) Greater London

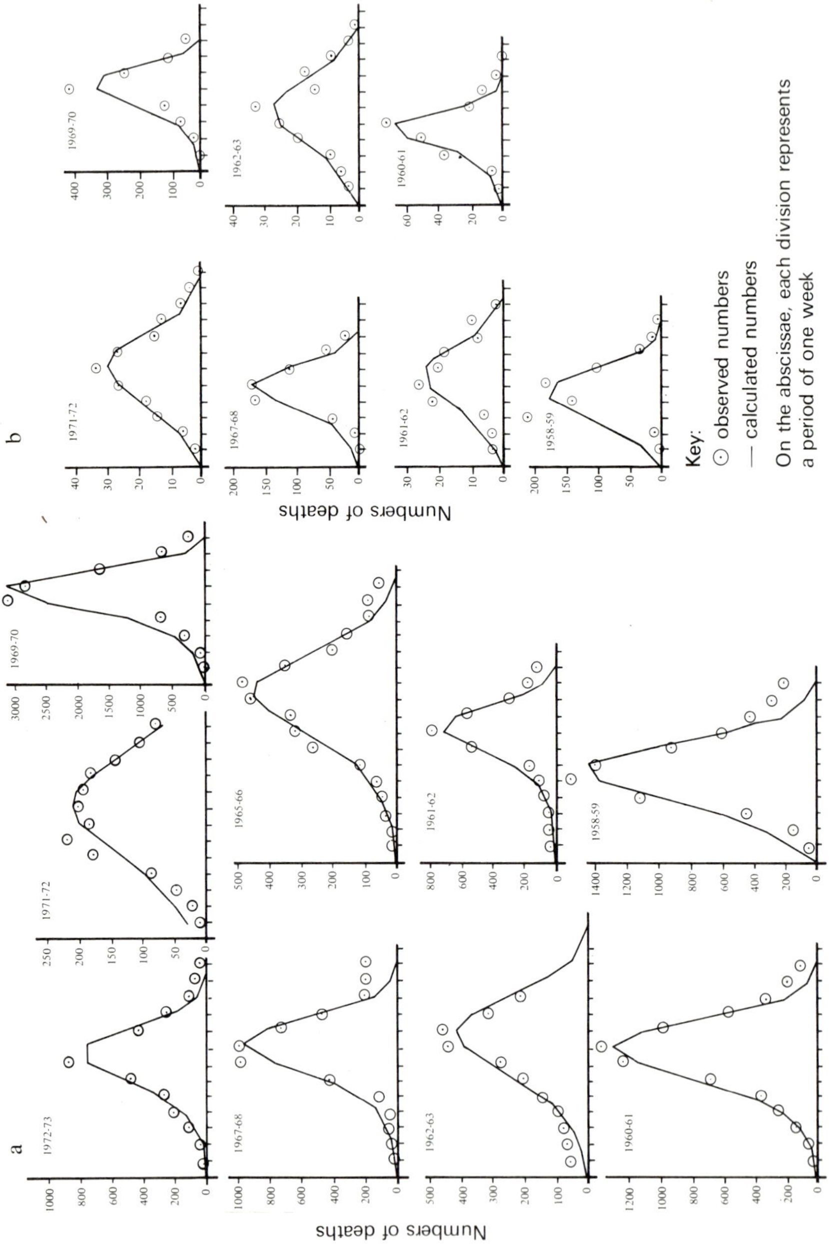

Values of $\alpha = \lambda S_o$ in England and Wales and Greater London, 1958-73

	England and Wales	*Greater London*
1958-59	5.2	5.6
1960-61	5.5	7.1
1961-62	6.5	5.0
1962-63	4.7	4.5
1965-66	4.5	—
1967-68	5.9	7.0
1969-70	7.7	7.7
1971-72	3.9	4.7
1972-73	5.7	—

Note: Years which were clearly unsuitable because of small numbers or bimodality are omitted.

serological information could be made available, cases accurately recorded, meteorological data collected, and the behavior of the disease in small groups such as schools and institutions observed, then the parameters of curves fitted to the epidemics might well become interpretable.

It would not be worthwhile to conduct a study solely for this purpose. But in communities which are being intensively studied there seems to be a good case for including mathematical modelling, either of the type outlined here or of the smaller-scale variety which will be described by Dr Elveback.

The stability of the infectivity parameter in the USSR experience makes it likely that their mathematical approach is more than a mere exercise in curve-fitting.

References

Bailey, N. T. J. (1975) *The mathematical theory of infectious diseases,* London: Griffin.

Baroyan, O. V., Rvachev, L. A., Basilevsky, U. V., Ermakov, V. V., Frank, K. D., Rvachev, M. A., and Shashkov, V. A. (1971) *Adv. Appl. Probab., 3,* 224-6.

Baroyan, O. V., Rvachev, L. A., and Ivannikov, Yu. G. (1977) *Modelling and prediction of influenza epidemics in the USSR,* Moscow: Gamaleia Institute (in Russian).

Kermack, W. O. and McKendrick, A. G. (1927) *Proc. Roy. Soc., A 115,* 700-21.

Spicer, C. C. (1979) *Brit. Med. Bull.,* Vol. 35, No. 1, 23-8.

Stuart-Harris, C. H., Franks, Z., and Tyrrell, D. A. J. (1950) *Brit. Med. J., 1,* 263-6.

Effects of weather on disease incidence and intensity

L. P. Smith

ABSTRACT

The main effects of weather on the epidemiology of foot-and-mouth disease, calf pneumonia, and some human infectious diseases are summarized. A short account is given of the successful simulation of the pattern of morbidity of acute bronchitis over seven years, using only meteorological data. Suggestions are made of ways in which the effects of weather on influenza incidence could usefully be analyzed.

Previous experience in considering the effect of weather on disease incidence in animals (foot-and-mouth disease and calf pneumonia) has led to the following deductions.

In foot-and-mouth disease:

1. Over 90% of the spread during the period prior to the introduction of movement restrictions was downwind during rain.

2. A decrease in an epidemic appeared to be related to a period of dry weather.

3. There was some suggestion that the incubation period was short at the beginning of an epidemic, but longer at later stages.

4. A major epidemic seemed to occur when there was a succession of coincidences in time of major virus output (usually the day before disease identification) and optimum weather conditions for spread.

In calf pneumonia:

1. Major problems of deaths were reported from calf-rearing houses which were situated in frost hollows.

2. Limited evidence suggested that single very cold nights were not sufficient to cause deaths. Two very cold nights, separated by the incubation period of the disease (16 days), appeared to be necessary for high mortality.

In regard to the spread of influenza, the following questions arise:

1. Can the virus be airborne over more than a limited distance, i.e. does it spread downwind?

2. If not, does the presence of a surface temperature inversion, such as occurs in foggy weather with little or no wind, increase the nose-level concentrations of emitted virus?

3. Does the occurrence of low temperatures at the beginning of the working day, implying a rapid change of ambient temperature on going outdoors, facilitate infection?

Influenza reaches its peak in winter. This suggests that one or more of the following weather factors may be significant:

1. Low outdoor temperature.
2. High outdoor relative humidity.
3. Very low indoor relative humidity.
4. Temperature inversions near ground level.

Examination of data provided by the Royal College of General Practitioners has shown that multiple regression analysis is possible, using the following weather factors:

for the febrile common cold	– previous minimum temperature
for febrile sore throat	– previous vapor pressure (implying low indoor relative humidity)
for acute bronchitis	– previous minimum temperature and high outdoor relative humidity
for otitis media	– previous minimum temperature.

Previous morbidity was taken as a measure of potential sources of infection, and previous morbidity over a period of 10-12 weeks was taken as a measure of the build-up of immunity. No trace of any immunity factor was found for bronchitis and sore throat. Some improvement in fit was found by using the square-root of the weekly or four-weekly morbidity data. Total correlation coefficients (on sets of independent data) were about 0.8. Partial correlation coefficients were about:

0.5 on an infection term

–0.35 on an immunity term

–0.5 on a weather factor.

The best fits were found in regard to bronchitis, with multiple correlations around 0.9. Using this regressive equation and starting with the morbidity for June 1967, thereafter using only weather data (and morbidity derived from weather data), it was possible to simulate the pattern of bronchitis outbreaks for the next seven years to a fair degree of accuracy. The closeness of fit is shown in the figure.

Attempts to use a similar approach to influenza data showed that minimum air temperatures up to two weeks previous to the morbidity data appeared to be significant. An immunity factor, calculated from running ten-week totals of morbidity, accounted for the decrease of an epidemic, but it was very difficult to obtain acceptable estimates of peak values of disease incidence, probably partly owing to the lack of information about the type or strain of virus.

I suggest that the problem could profitably be considered in stages:

1. Time of start of an epidemic.
2. Rate of increase.
3. Peak incidence.
4. Rate of decrease.

Evidence so far suggests that more detailed use of daily mimimum temperature data might be useful. The existence, and persistence, of surface temperature inversions could be important.

The search for repeated, periodic low temperatures might also be rewarding. For example, in the 1969-70 influenza outbreak, very cold nights (and early mornings) occurred every ten days or so for 50-60 days before the peak disease week. This did not happen in other years when the peak incidence was much lower.

Bibliography

Smith, L. P., and Hugh-Jones, M. E. (1969) The weather factor in foot-and-mouth epidemics, *Nature, 223,* 712-15.

Smith, L. P., ed. (1970) Weather and animal diseases, *World Meteorological Organization Technical Note, 113,* 19-27.

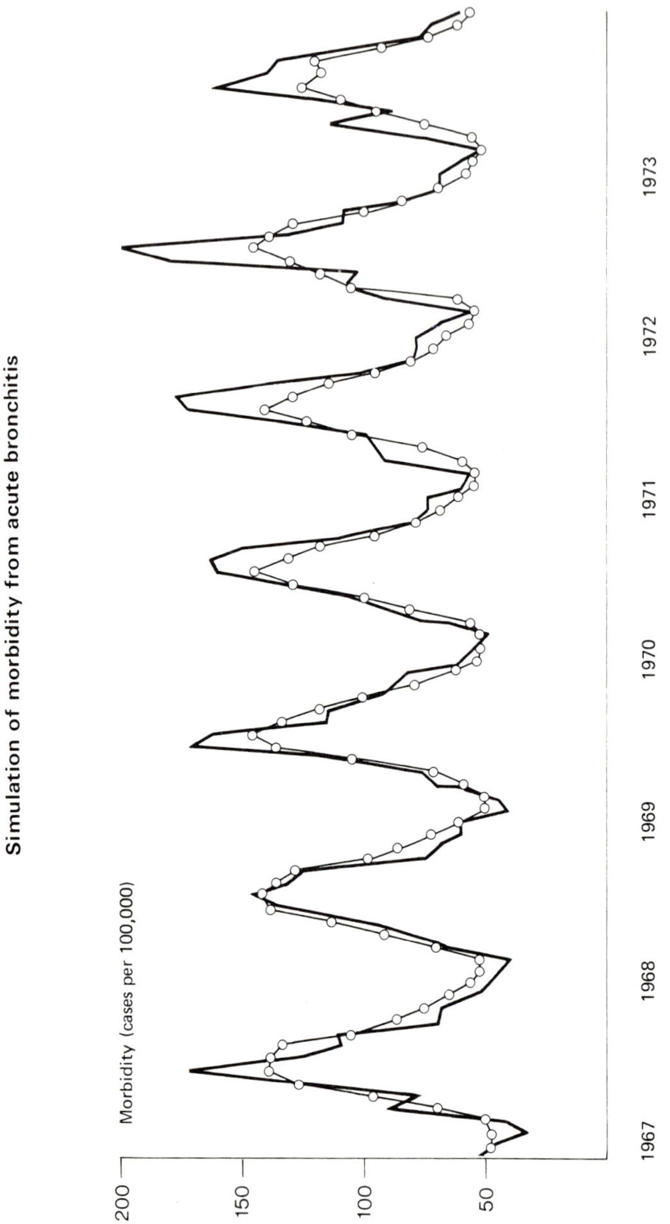

Comparison of the actual morbidity due to acute bronchitis in Britain, using 28-day data, with the simulated morbidity, calculated from the actual morbidity in June 1967 and thereafter using only the minimum air temperature and relative humidity data. Open circles indicate calculated values.

The speed of approach to peak morbidity in influenza epidemics

L. P. Smith

ABSTRACT

Analysis of the RCGP influenza data for the UK, on a weekly basis, shows that the peak incidence in an epidemic is highly correlated with the rate of increase in incidence, per 100,000 per week, in the initial stages. Attempts are made to identify this critical initial period by reference to the previous occurrence of mean weekly minimum air temperatures and to minimum air temperatures on individual nights. Reasonable accuracy is attained for the major epidemic years.

Data on the incidence of influenza in the UK, collected by the epidemic observation unit of the Royal College of General Practitioners (RCGP) since 1967, provide the number of new diagnoses per 100,000 inhabitants for each successive week. Examination of such data covering a period of eight years suggested that the rate of increase of this incidence in the initial stages of an epidemic is closely related to the maximum weekly incidence, or "peak morbidity". A search was therefore made for those critical weeks, previous to the peak, which would give the most reliable indication of the epidemic intensity. If these critical weeks could be identified from weather data, then an opportunity presented itself of forecasting the intensity of the subsequent epidemic.

1. Analysis of the initial stages of disease spread

If the week in which peak influenza incidence occurs be called "week 0", then, numbering backwards in time, the previous weeks can be called "week 1", "week 2", "week 3", etc.

Using the RCGP data for the UK, I calculated the average rate of increase of incidence per week, which can be termed the "morbidity speed". This was done over periods of three weeks (week 5 to week 3), four weeks (week 6 to week 3), and five weeks (week 7 to week 3), using Marvin's Method (see Annex). The formulae used were as follows:

(a) Given three successive weeks, with morbidities M_5, M_4, and M_3, respectively, then:

$$\text{"morbidity speed" } (MS_3) = \frac{2(M_3 - M_5)}{4}$$

(b) Given four successive weeks, with morbidities M_6, M_5, M_4, and M_3, respectively, then:

$$\text{"morbidity speed" } (MS_4) = \frac{3(M_3 - M_6) + (M_4 - M_5)}{10}$$

(c) Given five successive weeks, with morbidities M_7, M_6, M_5, M_4, and M_3, respectively, then:

$$\text{"morbidity speed" } (MS_5) = \frac{4(M_3 - M_7) + 2(M_4 - M_6)}{20}$$

The results are shown in Table 1 (the years being listed according to peak morbidity). They suggest that the peak intensity of the disease is strongly related to its pattern of development over the period 3 to 7 weeks previously.

While this may be useful in fitting an algebraic curve to the plot of disease incidence in any numerical model, it is so far useless for any simple prediction of peak intensity, as there is no means of knowing when "week 3" has been reached. To resolve this difficulty, it seemed reasonable to devise some criterion based on minimum air temperature. Data from Kew Observatory were analyzed for this purpose, assuming that the minimum temperatures at that site would act as reference points, not as representative values for the whole country. (The Observatory has since been closed, and a new source of data would have to be used for any future study.)

2. Use of mean weekly minimum air temperatures

The required critical week ("week 3") was assumed to be the fourth week in late autumn or early winter which had a mean weekly minimum air temperature of 3° C or less. The "morbidity speed" was calculated over periods of four and five weeks, ending with this assumed "week 3". The results are shown in Table 2.

TABLE 1

Correlation of peak morbidity with "morbidity speed" at different time intervals preceding the peak

Year	*Peak morbidity (per 100,000)*	*Morbidity speed over the weeks prior to week 3*		
		Weeks 5 to 3	*Weeks 6 to 3*	*Weeks 7 to 3*
1969-70	918	137.5	91.2	64.0
1972-73	520	74.5	53.8	39.2
1967-68	262	32.5	23.6	18.9
1971-72	222	0.3	23.9	23.5
1968-69	152	13.0	1.8	3.7
1973-74	121	3.5	7.0	3.3
1970-71	39	4.0	4.5	2.9
1966-67	24	−1.0	−0.6	0.4
Correlation with peak morbidity		0.98	0.99	0.975

The anomalies of the Christmas week, in which the reported incidence was clearly lower than expected, had to be accepted.

TABLE 2

Correlation of peak morbidity with "morbidity speed" at different time intervals preceding the estimated critical week, the latter being defined in terms of mean weekly minimum air temperatures

Year	*Peak morbidity (per 100,000)*	*Morbidity speed during weeks preceding critical week*		*Subsequent time to peak week*
		Preceding 4 weeks	*Preceding 5 weeks*	
1969-70	918	91.2	64.0	3 weeks
1972-73	520	50.4	55.8	1 week
1967-68	262	59.1	44.3	2 weeks
1971-72	222	1.9	1.3	10 weeks
1968-69	152	4.6	3.5	9 weeks
1973-74	121	0.4	0.4	16 weeks
1970-71	39	−1.1	1.1	1 week
1966-67	24	0.7	0.25	5 weeks
Correlation with peak morbidity		0.90	0.88	

This approach appears to identify the major and minor epidemics, but the timing in particular is unsatisfactory. The next attempt used the minimum air temperatures on individual nights, in the hope that these might give better results.

3. Use of minimum air temperatures on individual nights

The critical "week 3" was taken to be the week after that in which the 20th night with a minimum air temperature below 3° C had occurred. The results are shown in Table 3.

This is a definite improvement on the previous method of identification, and provides the basis for a possible forecast of epidemic peak three weeks ahead. The most misleading results are those for 1968-69 and 1973-74, and it is clear that the temperature factor has still to be correctly identified and specified.

TABLE 3

Correlation of peak morbidity with "morbidity speed" at different time intervals preceding the estimated critical week, the latter being defined in terms of minimum air temperatures on individual nights

Year	*Peak morbidity (per 100,000)*	*Morbidity speed during weeks preceding critical week*		*Subsequent time to peak week*
		Preceding 4 weeks	*Preceding 5 weeks*	
1969-70	918	91.2	64.0	3
1972-73	520	53.8	39.2	3
1967-68	262	23.6	18.9	3
1971-72	222	5.8	3.8	9
1968-69	152	−1.6	101.8	
1973-74	121	0.4	4.0	16
1970-71	39	3.5	4.0	2
1966-67	24	1.3	0.7	4
Correlation with peak morbidity		0.98	0.99	

4. Constant scrutiny of "morbidity speed" without access to temperature data

As long as the "morbidity speed" calculated from four weekly sets of disease data (MS_4) is less than ten, there is no evidence that the peak morbidity will exceed 50 per 100, 000. If MS_4 exceeds ten, however, the likely peak morbidity is correspondingly higher, as shown in Table 4.

Any deduction from this type of evidence becomes very misleading in the period just before the peak week, when the speed becomes very great, as shown in Table 5. This danger arises because we have no indication of the timing of the peak week from disease data alone.

Nevertheless, constant scrutiny of the "morbidity speed' could provide useful information, a rise to over 30 acting as a danger signal, and one to over 70 as an alarm.

Conclusions

The speed of epidemic spread in its early stages, and perhaps the rate of increase of such speed (its "acceleration"), deserves more careful analysis with a longer series of data. The present temperature criteria need to be improved by better interpretation. The behavior of the "morbidity speed" of the febrile common cold may give a lead in this

TABLE 4

Four-week "morbidity speed", likely peak morbidity, and subsequent time to peak

MS_4	*Likely peak morbidity (per 100,000)*	*Examples, and subsequent time in weeks to peak (in brackets)*
Over 10	Over 100	121(2); 152(8); 222(8); 263(4); 520(4); 918(4)
Over 20	Over 150	152(1); 222(7); 263(3); 520(4); 918(4)
Over 30	Over 200	222(5); 263(2); 520(3); 918(3)
Over 50	Over 260	262(2); 520(3); 918(3)
Over 70	Over 500	520(2); 918(3)
Over 90	Over 900	918(3)

respect, as this disease and influenza both seem to respond to the same type of weather.

TABLE 5

Peak morbidity and "morbidity speed" just before and during the peak week

Year	*Peak morbidity (per 100,000)*	*Morbidity speed up to week before peak*	*Morbidity speed (MS_4) at peak week*
1972-73	520	50.4	105.5
1969-70	918	229.4	215.6

Annex

If, with two sets of variables, the independent variables are equally spaced, then the regression equation between them can be found by simple arithmetic in Marvin's Method, as follows:

The dependent variables y_1, y_2, etc. are written in two columns, one down and one up, so that half the variables appear in each column. If the total number is odd, then the "center value" is written by itself at the bottom.

The left-hand column is subtracted from the right-hand column, giving differences $y_n - y_1$, $y_{n-1} - y_2$, etc.

These differences are then multiplied by weighting factors $n - 1$, $n - 3$, $n - 5$, etc. If the total number n is even, then the smallest weighting factor is 1; if n is odd, then the smallest factor is 0, which is then multiplied by the "center value" standing by itself at the foot of the two columns.

For example, when $n = 4$:

$y_4 - y_1$ multiplied by 3
$y_3 - y_2$ multiplied by 1

When $n = 5$:

$y_5 - y_1$ multiplied by 4
$y_4 - y_2$ multiplied by 2
y_3 multiplied by 0.

The weighted differences are then summed, giving a total, G.

The regression equation $y = a + bx$ is then given by:

$$a = M - \tfrac{1}{2}(n - 1)b$$
$$b = G \div S$$

where M is the mean of the dependent variables y_r and

$$S = \frac{(n - 1)(n)(n + 1)}{6}$$

For values of $n = 3$, 4, and 5, $S = 4$, 10, and 20, respectively.

Models of the temporal spread of epidemics (3)

K. Choi

ABSTRACT

The first stage in modelling the spread of an influenza epidemic is to accurately describe the observed phenomena (such as mortality or morbidity statistics) without assuming any underlying biological process. The second stage is to validate and improve models of the underlying biological process (such as mass-action models). The first stage is essential not only for the construction of realistic models, but also for forecasting the temporal spread of epidemics. Not much attention has been paid to the problem of describing the course of an epidemic dynamically and longitudinally.

As an example of such efforts, I shall describe a method of estimating the excess mortality due to an influenza epidemic in the USA. The method is currently used by the Centers for Disease Control (CDC) to monitor the pneumonia and influenza (P & I) deaths in 121 cities.

One way to describe the severity of an epidemic is to estimate the excess of P & I deaths over the number to be expected in the absence of an epidemic. However, there are several drawbacks to using the weekly number of P & I deaths as an indicator of influenza activity. Even though the CDC issued detailed reporting procedures, the degree and type of compliance by collaborators in the 121 cities vary widely. For example, we do not know the population pool in each city and its suburbs from which deaths are reported. Finally, the date of death as reported to the CDC is the one appearing on the death certificate, rather than the actual date of death. As a result, the CDC receives notification of deaths for only 3-5 days during a holiday week, but for 9-11 days during the week following a holiday week. If the ratio of the sum of P & I deaths to the total number of deaths from all causes is used as an indicator of influenza activity, problems such as vagaries in the reporting procedures, lack of clarity in defining the population at risk, and holiday effects are eliminated.

Previously, CDC used the regression method of Serfling (1963) to obtain the expected number of weekly P & I deaths. Serfling deleted the P & I deaths during the past epidemic periods, and fitted a regression equation from the past five-year data. The regression equation was used to forecast the expected P & I deaths for the coming year. The Serfling method tended to underestimate the expected P & I deaths, because data from epidemic weeks were omitted.

To overcome the defects of the regression method of forecasting expected P & I mortality, the CDC made the following three modifications:

–use of the P & I ratio rather than the observed number of deaths,

–replacement of P & I ratios for the epidemic periods with ratios forecast under the assumption of a no-epidemic activity, rather than deleting data from epidemic weeks,

–forecasting by the auto-regressive integrated moving average (ARIMA) model proposed by Box and Jenkins (1976). This is based on time-series analysis, utilizing the dynamic relationship among numbers of deaths in previous weeks to estimate expected deaths in subsequent weeks.

It was shown that the ARIMA model was approximately 50% more accurate than the regression model in forecasting the P & I ratio. The ARIMA model also revealed an underlying pattern in the P & I mortality data. The P & I mortality in the current week was estimated from that in the previous four weeks of the same year and the corresponding four weeks in the two previous years. Details are given by Choi and Thacker (1981).

Having established the expected P & I deaths, which is the base-line of mortality, the next step in our analysis is to construct a stochastic model for the temporal spread of epidemics by the superposition of the following two stochastic processes:

–constructing a point process model which triggers an epidemic according to the probability estimated from the past data and,

–given that an epidemic process is triggered, constructing an ARIMA model of the epidemic which is determined by the characteristics of the prevailing strain of influenza virus.

References

Box, G. E. P., and Jenkins, G. M. (1976) *Time series analysis, forecasting and control*, San Francisco: Holden Day.

TEMPORAL SPREAD (Choi)

Choi, K., and Thacker, S. B. (1981) An evaluation of influenza mortality surveillance, 1962-1979: (I) Time series forecasts of expected pneumonia and influenza deaths, (II) Percentage of pneumonia and influenza deaths as an indicator of influenza activity, *Amer. J. Epid. 113*, 3.

Serfling, R. E. (1963) Methods for current statistical analysis of excess pneumonia-influenza deaths, *Publ. Hlth Rep., 78*, 494-506.

Session II: Discussion of presentations by Bailey, Spicer, L. Smith, and Choi

Rapporteur: Fine

Tyrrell noted that a major virtue of working with applied mathematicians is that it prevents sloppy thinking. The process of model-building forces clarity of thought and argument.

L. Smith commented that this association with mathematical work is both difficult and rewarding for biological workers, in that many of them left mathematics at an elementary level.

Fine commented that Spicer's work involved fitting the model to data on entire epidemics, whereas the Russian work involved derivation of parameters on the basis of early epidemics, and comparison of predictions with "independent" data from later epidemics in other cities. It would be of interest to see how well the model predicted the latter part of UK epidemics after being fitted to data from the initial phase.

Bailey and Elveback both referred to current scepticism concerning certain claims for the Rvachev-Baroyan model, which some believed to be inadequately supported in publications.

Elveback enquired whether excess mortality trends were seen to move either east-west or north-south across the USA. It seems there is no clear evidence for a consistent trend in any direction.

Tyrrell asked in what circumstances weather data were likely to provide effective prediction of disease spread.

L. Smith commented that the cumulative effects of past weather provide far stronger predictive power than does current weather. For example, they provide a basis for predictions of potato blight and apple scab. Long-range predictions are most effective with reference to helminthic infections of animals, because weather affects the developmental stages of larvae, or the intermediate host of flukes, and this is reflected in incidence patterns several months later.

Tyrrell wondered how weather might provide a trigger for influenza epidemics.

L. Smith suggested that a sudden drop in temperature might take many people by surprise. They would get chilled because of inadequate clothing, and this could make them more susceptible.

Spicer considered that Hoyle and Wickramasinghe's book *Diseases from Space* should not be totally discounted, since it includes interesting data on the association of influenza with weather fronts.

L. Smith noted that weather fronts have been associated with odd psychological behavior and traffic accidents, but doubted whether they would affect influenza spread. He raised the possibility that weather factors might affect viral mutation rates.

Tyrrell pointed out that Lidwell's data from Newcastle suggested an association between common colds and either a fall in temperature or a rise in relative humidity.

Stuart-Harris observed that not all influenza outbreaks begin in winter. For example, Asian 'flu began in the UK in mid-summer, perhaps triggered by crowd assemblies at the onset of the football season.

Elveback recalled that the Tangipahoa epidemic in Louisiana also began in summer, in association with the opening of schools in that community.

J. Smith suggested that the Russian data do not imply a large weather effect, if the spread is effectively explained by transportation.

L. Smith replied that weather still might be of importance in triggering epidemics in the USSR. The Russian winter is uniformly severe, and its effects after initiation of an epidemic may be consistent throughout the country.

Tyrrell noted that the effect of weather is likely to be most clearly observed in situations where an infectious agent is constantly present in an area. If an agent is only intermittently present other, non-weather factors are likely to predominate.

J. Smith asked what were the implications of Choi's findings that three sine curves, with six-month, one-year, and three-year cycles, provide an excellent description of pneumonia and influenza mortality in the USA.

Choi noted that both auto-regression and spectral analyses produce the three-year cycle, but that this is less powerful than the other cycles. It may be that the six-month cycle takes care of the "wiggles", the one-year cycle takes care of the annual cycles, and the three-year cycle introduces a secular trend.

Bailey enquired whether the three-year cycle might reflect a susceptible "depletion – repletion" cycle, rather like the two-year pattern of measles, which is explained as reflecting the period necessary to build up a sufficient susceptible population for a subsequent epidemic.

Tyrrell suggested that more attention be paid to work on measles, in order to explain the underlying dynamics of influenza.

Fine described an analysis of weekly measles data from the UK, applying the simple discrete-time mass-action model. The expression discussed by Spicer can be simplified to:

$$C_{t+1} = C_t \cdot S_t \cdot \lambda_t$$

where C_t and S_t are numbers of cases and susceptibles at time *t*, and C_{t+1} is the number of cases one serial interval later. The λ_t is called different things by different authors, like "infectivity" or "force of infection" or "contact rate", but it is better to speak of it neutrally as a "transmission parameter", as the other terms have inappropriate and misleading implications. A simple rearrangement of this equation gives:

$$\frac{C_1}{C_0} = S_0\lambda = \alpha_0$$

$S_0\lambda$ or α_0 is the parameter derived at the outset of epidemics in the Russian model. It is analogous to the "basic reproduction rate" or the "transmission-to-case ratio" or the "number of effective contacts per case", in the early part of an epidemic. It is interesting that Spicer found this parameter had a range of about 4.5 to 7.7 for influenza epidemics in the UK.

The "transmission parameter" λ_t can be derived directly as:

$$\lambda_t = \frac{C_{t+1}}{S_t \cdot C_t}$$

if data are available on numbers of cases in successive serial intervals and numbers of susceptibles. This has been done for measles, revealing that the parameter changes markedly with season, with a dramatic rise at the onset of each school term. This indicates that schools are more important than weather in determining measles patterns. It would be of interest to explore such analyses for influenza, but unfortunately the appropriate data are not available.

Elveback noted that several participants have graduate students, and that this meeting could prove valuable if it came up with suggestions as to useful topics for higher-degree student research projects.

Abstract of discussion

1. Modelling is a healthy, if sometimes strenuous, exercise for biomedical scientists.

2. More evidence is needed of the predictive value of the Rvachev-Baroyan influenza model.

3. The relationship between weather patterns and influenza is not understood. Certain changes or cumulative effects of weather might trigger epidemics.

4. Some influenza epidemics seem to have been triggered by social aggregation, with little or no evidence of weather effects.

5. Six, 12, and 36-month cycles in pneumonia-influenza mortality may reflect seasonal cycles, susceptible depletion-repletion cycles, and secular trends, on top of statistical artifacts in data.

6. The α parameter in the Rvachev-Baroyan and Spicer models is analogous to the basic reproductive rate concept, and measures the average number of transmissions per case in the early phase of an epidemic.

7. Measles cycles are determined more by dates of school terms than by weather patterns. This may have implications for influenza.

Session III

Models of family and small community spread

Elveback

Bailey

Models of family and small community spread (1)

L. R. Elveback

ABSTRACT

A discrete-time stochastic model for influenza immunization studies is summarized. A simulated population of 1,000 was divided into four age groups, with subgroup mixing in families, neighborhoods, pre-school play-groups, and school, as well as total community mixing. The infective process involves the probabilities of infection following contact (relative susceptibility), of illness following infection, and of withdrawal following illness, and the response pattern following vaccination. Latent and infectivity periods (2-4 days and 3-6 days, respectively), and the relative infectiousness to others, are random variables. Output is in terms of the distribution of epidemic size and age-specific attack rates.

I shall review briefly the stochastic simulation model (Elveback et al., 1976). This study was a team effort involving Dr John Fox, virologist and immunologist, Dr Eugene Ackerman, mathematical biologist and computer scientist, and myself.

We simulated a small suburban community with a highly-structured population of 1,000 people, in four age groups: pre-school, school, young adults, and older adults. Each person belonged to one of 254 families, and to one of 50 clusters representing neighborhoods and other mixing groups. The pre-school children each belonged to one of 30 play-groups, and the school-age children attended a single school. In addition, all individuals mixed in the total community. In each of these 336 mixing groups, an age-specific contact rate could be selected. We used a discrete time-interval of one day.

Characteristics of individuals

Each of the 1,000 individuals was characterized in terms of age, family, other mixing groups, relative susceptibility (probability of infection if contact occurred), and response pattern if immunized.

Random variables

There are a number of random variables, each with assignable distribution functions. The latent period is 1, 2, or 3 days (mean 1.9) and the infectivity period is 3 to 6 days (mean 4.1).

The pathogenicity, or probability of illness if infection occurred, was taken as 0.67 for all ages. The probability of withdrawal to the home if illness occurred was age-specific, being highest in pre-school children and lowest in adults. The number of days of circulation in mixing groups prior to withdrawal to the home was 0, 1, or 2 days, with probabilities depending on age. Relative infectiousness, or the probability of transmitting infection if contact with a susceptible occurred, was taken as unity for those who become ill, and as 0.5 for those who are infectious but not ill. The relative infectiousness was given several different distribution functions in the "superspreader" studies.

Each day, the computer cycles through the remaining susceptibles to determine their infection fate for that day. For each susceptible individual, it determines the number of cases in each of his mixing groups, the relative infectiousness of each case, and the contact rate of the susceptible individual in each mixing group.

The probability that individual i becomes infected on a given day is computed as $1 - e^{-Z_i}$

$$\text{where} \qquad Z_i = S_i \sum_{g=1}^{G} p_{ig} \sum_{c=1}^{C_g} \theta_c$$

where,

S_i = relative susceptibility of individual i

G = the number of his mixing group

P_{ig} = his contact rate in mixing group g

θ_c = relative infectiousness of infectious case c

C_g = the number of cases in mixing group g.

The outcome is determined by generation of a random number. The model is sufficiently general to serve for any agent which spreads from person to person.

The contact rates were determined by trial and error to fit several published results (Carey et al., 1958; Chin et al., 1960; Davis et al., 1970; Dunn et al., 1959; Jordan et al., 1958) for both Asian and Hong Kong epidemics. The published results in each case consisted of age-specific illness attack rates, and age-specific secondary illness attack rates in families with schoolchildren. These attack rates differed in different reports. We selected an appropriate range for each, and feel that the

FIGURE 1

Influenza model: possible course of infection for each susceptible individual

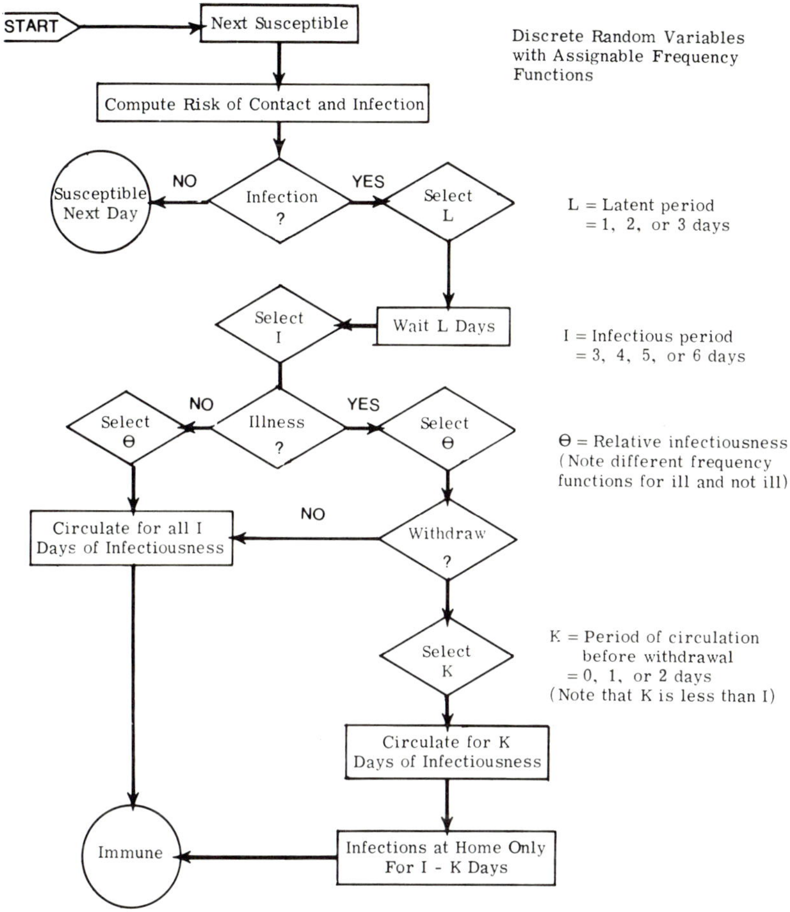

values we selected are adequate to serve as background against which to measure the effectiveness of various vaccine strategies.

The results can be described in several ways, which are illustrated in Figures 2-6.

The table shows age-specific attack rates for illness and for infection. Similar tables can be constructed for age-specific secondary attack rates (SAR). Although our results gave an adequate fit to the

Baseline attack rates (percentage) in Asian influenza epidemics

Age group	Families with school-children	Families without school-children	Total population	
	Illness	*Illness*	*Illness*	*Infection*
Pre-school children	40	29	35	54
School-children	64		64	91
Young adults	26	17	23	35
Older adults	15	10	13	20

FIGURE 2

Epidemic curves, as shown by the number of new infections each day. The Asian curve reflects an explosive outbreak in the schools, as compared with the slower progress of the Hong Kong epidemics.

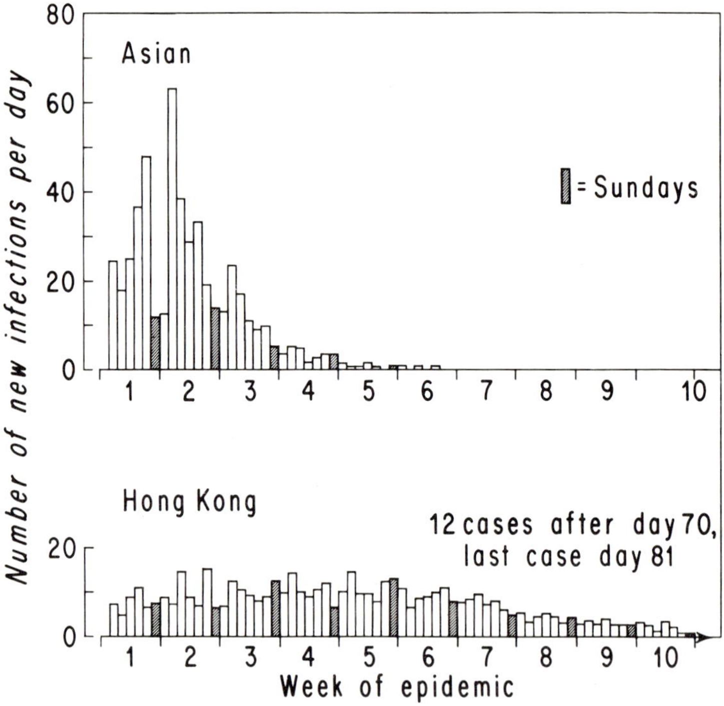

FIGURE 3

The distribution of epidemic size

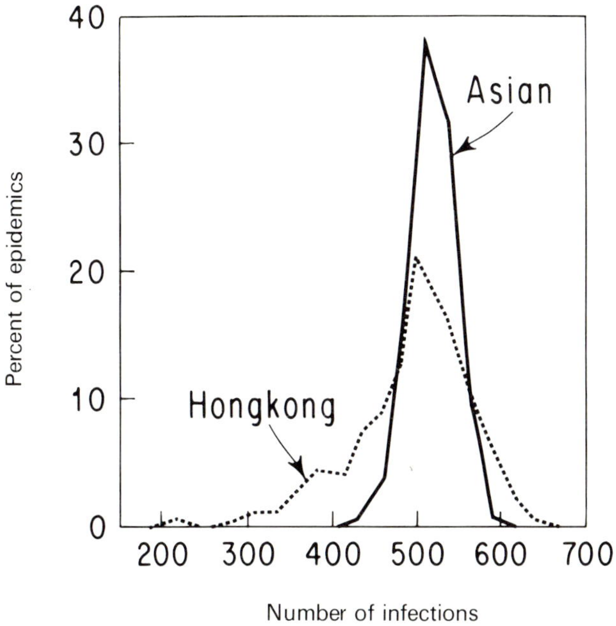

The curve for the Asian virus is based on 500 epidemics. That for the Hong Kong virus is based on 200 epidemics, since the computer time required was longer.

published reports, we do not consider these SAR results particularly useful in this epidemic situation. In the case of the Asian virus we found that, if we set the family contact rates to zero, the resulting SARs were approximately one-half of those found when infections occurred within the family. This points up the difficulty of distinguishing between cases acquired through family or non-family contacts.

The cost of running this program, together with all the sub-routines to store family data and compute SARs, was about $120 per set of 100 epidemics. If the SARs are eliminated, as I feel they should be when we are modelling an epidemic, the cost is halved. If the random variables are all eliminated and means are used, the cost is halved again, to $30 per set of 100 epidemics.

FIGURE 4

The epidemic curves for the Asian virus in schoolchildren, others, and the total population, as shown by the percentage of infectious persons each day

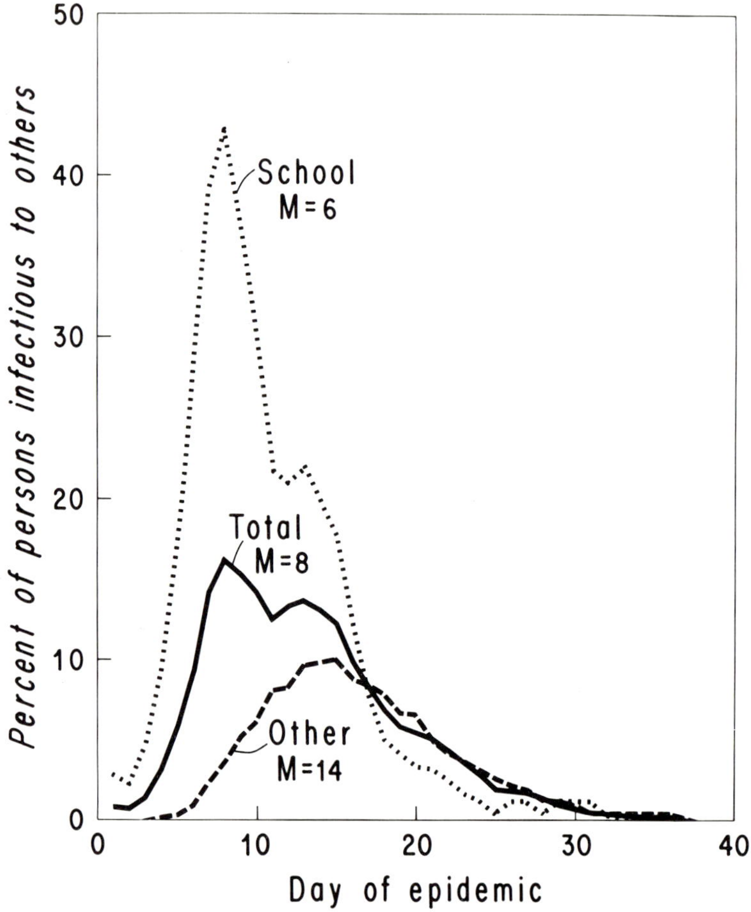

A graduate student is now engaged in re-working the model so that it will run at greatly reduced cost on a minicomputer. This will give us new potential for sensitivity studies.

FIGURE 5

Differences in epidemic size resulting from the vaccination of various percentages of schoolchildren at 28 days or more before the virus invades the community (allowing time for maximum immunity to develop in those vaccinated)

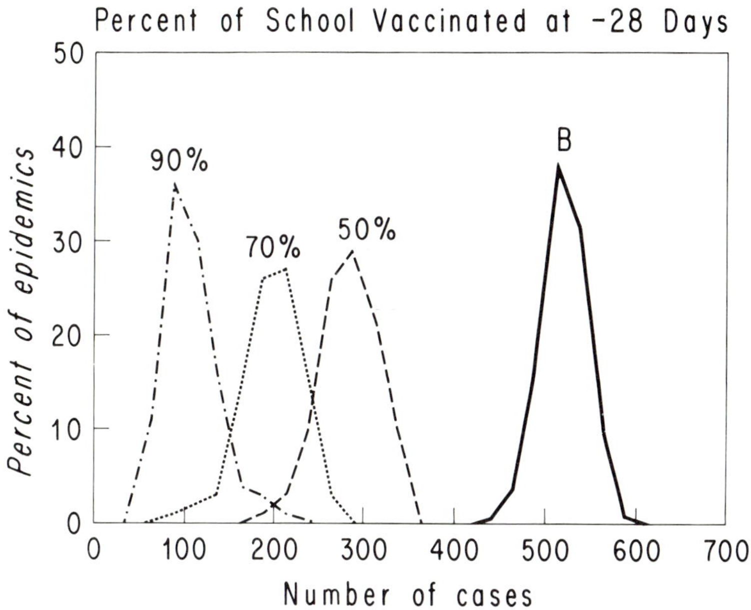

B = baseline (no vaccination).

Longini et al. (1978) have mapped our model onto a deterministic model which eliminates the population structuring and maintains only age, relative susceptibility, and relative infectiousness by age, and in which the latent and infectious periods are constant. Using the results of the simulation studies, they found contact rates which adequately reproduced our earlier results. The program runs very rapidly on a minicomputer, and solves the cost problem. For a new virus, for which simulation results are not available, this program would be dependent, as we were in our earlier work, on published results. Longini is currently working on Fox's family surveillance results, which cover non-epidemic periods and are based on illness, virus isolation, and serology.

FIGURE 6

Differences in epidemic size resulting from the vaccination of 70% of schoolchildren at 28, 10, and 3 days before the epidemic begins

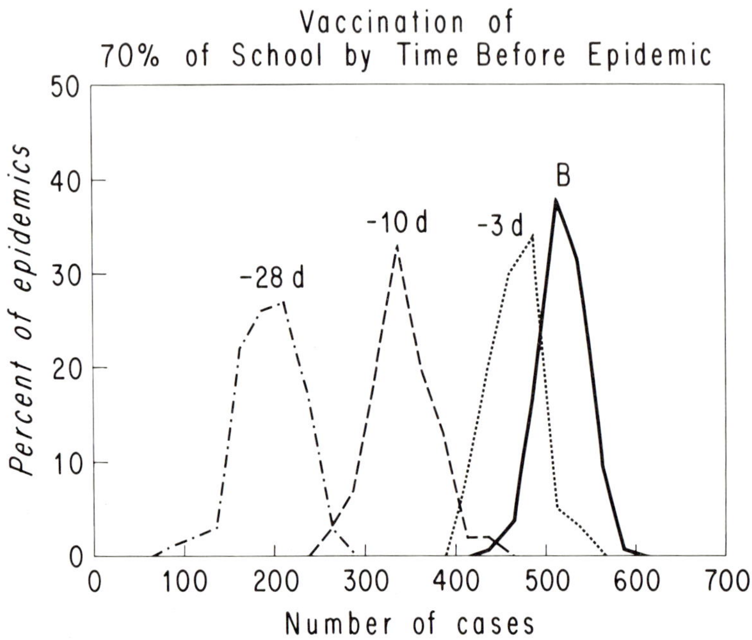

References

Carey, D. E. et al. (1958) Community-wide epidemic of Asian strain influenza: clinical and subclinical illness among school children, *J. Amer. med. Ass.*, *167*, 1459-63.

Chin, T. D. Y. et al. (1980) Morbidity and mortality characteristics of Asian strain influenza, *Pbl. Hlth Rep.*, *75*, 149-58.

Davis, L. E. et al. (1970) Hong Kong influenza: the epidemiologic features of a high school family study analyzed and compared with a similar study during the 1957 Asian influenza epidemic, *Amer. J. Epid.*, *92*, 240-7.

Dunn, F. L. et al. (1959) Epidemiologic studies of Asian influenza in a Louisiana parish, *Amer. J. Hyg.*, *70*, 351-71

Elveback, L. R. et al. (1976) An influenza simulation model for immunization studies, *Amer. J. Epid.*, *103*, 152-65.

Jordan, W. S., Jr. et al. (1958) A study of illness in a group of Cleveland families. XVII. The occurrence of Asian influenza, *Amer. J. Hyg.*, *68*, 190-212.

Longini, I. M., Jr. et al. (1978) An optimization model for influenza A epidemics, *Math. Biosci.*, *38*, 141-57.

Models of family and small community spread (2)

N. T. J. Bailey

ABSTRACT

If data are available from small groups like households, it may be possible to fit and test models in detail and to estimate parameters of epidemiological importance. The incorporation of stochastic elements is essential, and may be important even in studying such phenomena as fade-out in populations as large as 250,000.

The so-called 'chain-binomial' type of model can be successfully fitted to measles data, provided that allowance is made for variation between households in the chance of infection. More elaborate models can also be adequately fitted to measles data, involving a variable latent period after infection followed by an extended infectious period. Some applications have also been made to household data on influenza. On the whole it seems as though such micro-models are appropriate, but some of the studies are not entirely convincing.

In principle, micro-modelling can be used to estimate some of the consequences of public health interventions, such as immunization, showing the specific effects on the chance of infection, the recovery rate, etc. Family studies also need to be more closely linked with broader community studies. Progress has been made in specific applications of stochastic simulation modelling to influenza, and this has considerable bearing on the effects of flexible immunization routines and variable vaccine response patterns.

Further work is urgently needed in developing models that can take account of the special characteristics of influenza, notably antigenic drifts and shifts.

1. General considerations

The study of small community groups, such as school classes and individual households, permits a more detailed examination to be made of a variety of epidemiological hypotheses. If models can be successfully fitted to data at this relatively disaggregated level, then a degree of confidence in them can be built up. This has implications both for the epidemiological understanding of mechanisms of disease transfer between individuals, and for broad population phenomena of direct relevance to possible public health interventions, which we shall be looking at in other sessions.

Because of the small numbers in family-sized groups, it is essential to take probability variations into account, i.e. so-called "stochastic" models must be used. When an infection is introduced into a family it might lead to one of many different patterns of spread, varying from no further cases after the initial one to infection of the whole group at risk. Careful statistical analysis of data on a sufficiently large number of families allows one to estimate the basic parameters, e.g. infection rates or recovery rates, calculate standard errors, and test goodness-of-fit between the assumptions made and the data observed.

In large community groups, and particularly in towns or cities, we might expect deterministic approaches to be adequate, at least as a first approximation. However, in some types of analysis probability considerations appear to be important even in quite large populations. Thus in population studies by Bartlett (1957, 1960) of disease fade-out for measles in cities of different sizes, certain stochastic aspects had important effects even in populations of about 250,000.

It follows that a good understanding of the spread of disease in small groups may have important repercussions for the population dynamics of larger groups. In particular, there may be consequences for the choice of control strategies, such as vaccination, isolation, or specific treatments.

2. Specific models for household groups

As early as 1928, Reed and Frost in the USA were using a very simplified kind of model in which there was a fixed incubation period followed by a very short period of infectiousness, supposed for simplicity to be contracted to a single point. A slightly different variant was put forward in the UK by Greenwood, in 1931. It could easily be shown that these models led to the occurrence of distinct generations of cases, each having a certain binomial distribution. Hence the term 'chain-binomial' models. The models worked moderately well for family data on measles, but significant chi-squares were obtained in detailed analyses. To begin with, satisfactory fits could be obtained only when the distribution of the *total* number of cases per family was examined. I later showed that acceptable goodness-of-fit tests could be achieved with a heterogeneity assumption, in which the probability of infection under specified conditions varied between households in a way that could be estimated from the data. A detailed review of this whole subject is given by Bailey (1975).

More detailed analyses of the actual observed time-intervals between successive cases in a large number of very small families, e.g. two or three susceptibles, enabled finer distinctions to be made. It could be assumed that following infection there was a variable latent period, after which an extended infectious period occurred. This involved at least four parameters. Applications were made to appropriate measles data and the relevant parameters estimated. Satisfactory agreement between theory and data was obtained for families of both two and three susceptibles. Satisfactory results were also obtained for limited data on infective hepatitis in families of three individuals. For larger groups, the analysis becomes progressively more difficult and there are many unsolved problems.

3. Applications to influenza

Most of the work on chain-binomial approaches and their various extensions has been carried out on measles data. But a number of authors have made limited applications to chicken-pox, mumps, the common cold, infectious hepatitis, etc.

A small amount of work on the use of chain-binomial models for household data on influenza has already been undertaken by Hope Simpson and Sutherland (1954), Yamamoto (1959), Sugiyama (1960, 1961), Owaka et al. (1971), etc. Not all of these studies were entirely convincing. But on the whole it is clear that an appropriate stochastic model is essential for analyzing family data, and more efforts are required in developing methods to take account of the special characteristics of influenza, including the occurrence of antigenic drifts and shifts.

As already mentioned, the analysis of micro-epidemics in small family groups offers possibilities of estimating parameters of epidemiological importance. It also permits an assessment of the consequences, at this level, of public health interventions like immunization: e.g. what are the effects on the chance of infection or the recovery rate?

It is also desirable to link such family studies with broader community-level models, in order that better use can be made of the available knowledge. Some progress in building such bridges has already been achieved with the stochastic simulation modelling of Elveback et al. (1976), which is specifically geared to influenza. In particular, this modelling takes into account flexible immunization routines and variable vaccine response patterns. But further work is required on estimating parameters from individual communities, and on investigating the sensitivity of conclusions to uncertainties in the assumptions. Dr Elveback, together with her co-workers, has already embarked on a number of investigations of this kind, and she will supply appropriate details in her own presentation.

References

Bailey, N. T. J. (1975) *The mathematical theory of infectious diseases*, London: Griffin.

Bartlett, M. S. (1957) Measles periodicity and community size, *J. Roy. Statist. Soc.*, Ser. A, *120*, 48-70.

Bartlett, M. S. (1960) The critical community size for measles in the United States, *J. Roy. Statist. Soc.*, Ser. A, *123*, 37-44.

Elveback, L. R., Fox, J. P., Ackerman, E., Langworth, A., Boyd, M., and Gatewood, L. (1976) An influenza simulation model for immunization studies, *Amer. J. Epid.*, *103*, 152-65.

Hope Simpson, R. E. and Sutherland, I. (1954) Does influenza spread within the household?, *Lancet*, *i*, 721-6.

Owaka, K., Sakamoto, K., and Tanaka, H. (1971) An epidemiological study on the incubation period of influenza, *Jap. J. Hyg.*, *26*, 264-7 (in Japanese).

Sugiyama, H. (1960) Some statistical contributions to the health sciences, *Osaka City Med. J.*, *6*, 141-58.

Sugiyama, H. (1961) Some statistical methodologies for epidemiological research of medical sciences, *Bull. Int. Statist. Inst.*, *38* (3), 137-51.

Yamamoto, K. (1959) A theoretical epidemiological study on the mode of infection of influenza in the household, *J. Osaka City Med. Center*, *9*, 2179-90.

Session III: Discussion of presentations by Elveback and Bailey

Rapporteur: Choi

Tyrrell asked what factors and what community sizes should be considered in modelling.

Bailey replied that three factors should be considered: virus properties affecting transmission, environmental qualities affecting transmission, and host determinants of immunity. He added that, in Bruce Hammond's model for a community of 200 people, affinity subgrouping by social group did not improve the accuracy of the model. Bartlett has shown that stochastic models are valid for populations up to a quarter of a million. In smaller populations an epidemic starts but soon dies out, whereas in a larger population it is sustained. These "threshold" population sizes may be insensitive to spatial distributions.

Spicer added that stochastic elements enter into models when the community is only just large enough to maintain the virus in non-epidemic periods. In larger communities, the virus will always be present. In smaller ones, it will always die out and only be reintroduced by immigration of new cases.

It would be interesting to analyze influenza data as Bartlett did for measles data, since the basic parameters are about the same for the two diseases.

Fine pointed out that there are deterministic models (e.g. Yorke et al., 1979) which explain why measles eventually dies out in a small community. Thus it is not clear that stochastic models are any "better" than deterministic ones as far as the extinction issue is concerned.

L. Smith observed that, in modelling, a fit which is based on a logical set of assumptions is more important that a simple curve fit.

Choi argued that stochastic models are not necessarily better than deterministic ones, but are often more realistic.

Griffiths pointed out that a model should only be as realistic as is necessary for its intended use.

Tyrrell noted that deterministic and stochastic models are complementary, rather than mutually exclusive.

J. Smith and Tyrrell both felt that it might be easier to model epidemics of influenza B, because only people under a certain age are susceptible and less antigenic drift occurs than among A strains. They suggested it might be worthwhile to study influenza B epidemics in residential schools, where serological data and virus isolations can easily be obtained. Hammond's model fits well for the Tristan da Cunha data, but does not fit John Kendall's Epsom college data, possibly because the college was not a closed community.

Bailey and Spicer pointed out that a school epidemic is a complex phenomenon. There are many interactions among the students, as well as contacts with staff and delivery men, etc. from outside, and there is no averaging effect such as occurs in a large community.

J. Smith suggested that, since kindergartens have attack rates often greater than 50%, they might be good for modelling.

Stuart-Harris observed that there are few good laboratory data for children under five years of age, and that modelling of schools is a challenge.

Tyrrell asked what statisticians could do about modelling for those rare individuals who are superspreaders. A few superspreaders among a large number of children can cause epidemics to take off rapidly.

Elveback replied that a wide variability of infectivity is known to exist among infectives, but it is not known how to measure it.

Spicer pointed out that we do not need to postulate superspreaders in order to explain the explosiveness of school epidemics. It could be explained as a consequence of a large group size (threshold theorem) in the Kermack-McKendrick model.

Tyrrell stated that a family might not be a good place to model for superspreaders, and they could perhaps be better studied among passengers travelling by air.

Elveback asked what kinds of observations were needed in order to incorporate superspreaders in models.

L. Smith asked whether anyone had measured the virus content of air, and what weather conditions were conducive to increased viral activity.

Tyrrell replied that the rate of inactivation of influenza virus is lowest in cool, dry air. Air has been sampled in the vicinity of cases of respiratory disease, but the concentration was clearly very low and the results have not been related to the temperature and humidity of the air. However, no work has been done to link stability of the airborne virus with the transmission parameter (λ).

Fine suggested that, in modelling, we should relate λ in a large population model to parameters in a family model. He commented that the secondary attack rate is still a useful measure of infectiousness. Identification of primary, secondary, and tertiary cases of influenza is difficult because of the short and variable incubation period. However, family studies could be valuable using a large number of families, and superspreaders might be revealed by a bimodality of secondary attack rates or within-family "probabilities of effective contact".

J. Smith said he was still intrigued with the idea of modelling epidemics in school communities having high clinical attack rates. He asked why such modelling was difficult. Was it because the ratio of clinical to subclinical infection in schools is higher than in the population as a whole? Does the virus change its properties in such situations? If so, a simple model might not fit the data for school epidemics.

Tyrrell replied that a change in the virus is possible, on the grounds that strains which change in different situations would be expected to survive better.

Fine pointed out another difficulty in modelling school epidemics: the schools studied may not represent a random sample, since the ones selected are often those with higher attack rates.

Elveback added that some schools have an illness attack rate of 20-30%, whereas in others it may be as high as 80-90%. Moreover, even in the same school the attack rate varies from time to time. An illness attack rate of 80% implies that the pathogenicity (percentage of infections resulting in illness) is not less than 80%, which is much higher than the 50% quoted as average by Stuart-Harris. A higher pathogenicity in children seems reasonable, considering their more limited experience with previous influenza viruses.

Fine and Spicer both pointed out that high attack rates could be explained by a Reed-Frost type hypothesis. If the number of initial susceptibles were larger than a critical size, then epidemics would take off rapidly and the resulting attack rates would be high.

Fine pointed out that there are important similarities between the two major influenza models, of Elveback and Fox on the one hand, and of Rvachev and Baroyan on the other. Each considers the population as being divided into subunits (in the Elveback model these are called social groups, whereas in the Rvachev model they are called cities), and virus transmission occurs both within and between these subunits at specified rates. A superficial difference occurs because the Rvachev model is based upon the simple mass-action equation: $C_{t+1} = C_t \cdot S_t \cdot r$, whereas the Elveback model uses a derivative of the Reed-Frost equation: $C_{t+1} = S_t(1 - (1 - p)^{C_t})$. But these two formulations can be shown to be virtually identical (see background paper). Indeed, these two models might actually be considered as two expressions of the same underlying structure, and it is possible that Longini's condensed version could apply to the Rvachev model as well as to that of Elveback.

Abstract of discussion

1. Models of the spread of influenza should take into consideration virus properties and environmental qualities affecting transmission, host determinants of immunity, and population size.

2. Stochastic models are needed to complement deterministic ones.

3. Modelling epidemics in schools, which often have a high attack rate, is a worthwhile challenge.

4. Models which include superspreaders should be constructed.

5. The transmission parameter λ in a large population model should be related to parameters in a family model, such as the secondary attack rate.

Session IV

Relationship of parameters to the real world

Bailey

Tyrrell

Relationship of parameters to the real world (1)

N. T. J. Bailey

ABSTRACT

Realistic models for a specific disease must be based on agreement between statisticians and epidemiologists, with regard to overall structure and specific flow-rates between compartments. Relevant parameters must be estimated from appropriate data. Models must be properly checked out and validated, e.g. by generating verifiable predictions.

Satisfactory models must incorporate the major epidemiological states considered of greatest relevance to specific situations under examination. Typical items are listed. Similarly, all relevant parameters must be incorporated, dealing with a variety of clinical, epidemiological, demographic, economic, and other factors. Again, typical items are listed.

Proper statistical analysis should be undertaken whenever possible, including parameter estimation, calculation of standard errors, testing of goodness-of-fit, and comparison of predictions with observations.

Many of these ideal requirements cannot be achieved in practice, at least to begin with. Therefore a priori *assumptions must be made about both model structure and parametric values. Such problems can be handled by the judicious use of* sensitivity analysis, *and more attention to this approach is needed.*

In addition, special efforts should be made to achieve the minimum model complexity required for practical efficiency. An appropriate balance must be found between the conflicting requirements of realism and tractability.

1. Introduction

In order to achieve realistic models, we first need to have agreement on an appropriate general structure. Thus, in discussions between epidemiologists and statisticians on the development of a model for a specific infectious disease, it is usual for the relevant epidemiological states to be debated first. Typically, a consensus is first arrived at, in which there is a tentative flow-chart, the compartments of which represent epidemiological states like 'susceptibles', 'infectious persons', 'carriers', etc.

The next step is to consider the rates of flow between the compartments, involving such parameters as infection rate, length of latent period, recovery rate, etc. In order to represent real epidemic processes, these parameters must somehow be estimated and given specific numerical values.

A set of compartments, with the appropriate rates of flow, then constitutes the essential model. The latter's general behavior in time can be described by a set of differential equations or difference equations. These equations can be manipulated by mathematical methods, or by suitably chosen computer calculations, in order to derive the logical consequences of the assumptions made. Such models have to be properly checked out and validated, e.g. by showing that they can generate verifiable predictions. If they fail to do this satisfactorily, they must be rejected or at least modified, and the process repeated. For further discussion of this whole subject, see Bailey, Session II above (p. 127).

Listed below are some typical epidemiological states that may need to be incorporated into an infectious disease model, along with various factors that may also have to be included by using appropriately chosen parameters.

2. Epidemiological states

The following list is of course only illustrative, and is in no way complete. What is appropriate to any particular situation must be decided according to the circumstances.

—susceptibles

—infected individuals in a latent state

—infected individuals who are infectious

—dead persons

—individuals who have recovered and are immune

—individuals with natural immunity

—individuals in different age groups

—individuals with different degrees of susceptibility or infectiousness

—carriers.

3. Parameters

Again, only a partial list can be given. But in most models there are many more parameters than compartments.

- —contact rate ('physical' contact)
- —susceptibility of susceptibles
- —infectiousness of infectious individuals
- —probability of 'adequate contact'
- —length of latent period
- —parameters describing distribution of latent period (e.g. mean, standard deviation, etc.)
- —length of infectious period
- —parameters describing distribution of infectious period
- —demographic parameters, e.g. birth rates, death rates, migration rates
- —rate of loss of immunity
- —virological, serological, immunological parameters
- —parameters relating to spatial or geographic structure
- —climatic parameters
- —costs and benefits
- —effects of drug treatments
- —effects of immunization.

4. Statistical problems

This is a suitable point at which to draw attention to a variety of statistical problems associated with modelling. These include the use of *a priori* estimates of parameters, the estimation of parameters from data (e.g. by maximum likelihood), the calculation of standard errors, the testing of models by goodness-of-fit tests, the comparison of predictions with actual observed events, etc.

5. Sensitivity analysis

In many cases the values of certain parameters may have to be guessed, or at least based on informed professional judgements. This leads to important questions of how uncertainties in the assumptions of a model may be reflected in uncertainties about the conclusions. The appropriate approach is that of *sensitivity analysis*. While this is used extensively in control engineering and physics, examples of epidemiological applications are relatively uncommon.

A recent publication, however, examined a typhoid fever model with nine compartments and 25 parameters (Bailey and Duppenthaler, 1980). Sensitivity analysis, using a statistical mode of presentation easily understood in epidemiological terms, showed that typical conclusions about the endemic levels were sensitive to only four of the 25 parameters.

Sensitivity to possible changes in model structure can also be investigated. Subsequent work on the typhoid model showed that the nine-compartment model could be reduced to five compartments with little loss of accuracy.

The use of such approaches shows how to reduce model complexity to the minimum required for usable, practical efficiency. It also helps to deal with the perennial conflict between realism and tractability: a highly complex model may be theoretically closer to reality, but it cannot be reliably handled by mathematical or computational techniques, nor can the multitude of parameters be satisfactorily estimated by any available data. Simple models, on the other hand, may be easy to analyze but are often regarded as unrealistic. An appropriate balance of conflicting requirements has to be found.

Reference

Bailey, N. T. J. and Duppenthaler, J. (1980) Sensitivity analysis in the modelling of infectious disease dynamics, *J. Math. Biol.*, *10*, 113-31.

Relationship of parameters to the real world (2)

D. A. J. Tyrrell

ABSTRACT

Epidemics of colds on Tristan da Cunha were studied for five years. A modified Kermack-McKendrick model could be fitted to the data from the epidemics, provided that different parameters were used. Records of clinical symptoms suggest that the epidemics were due to different viruses. Some influenza viruses do not spread in human populations. It would be of interest to study those laboratory properties of influenza viruses which might determine their ability to spread and contribute to λ*. The numbers of susceptibles have been estimated from serological data in Sheffield, and suggest that epidemics die out when one-half to three-quarters of the population have become resistant to the circulating virus.*

The island of Tristan da Cunha, situated in mid-Atlantic between Argentina and South Africa, is inhabited by little more than 200 individuals, who live in a small village and are visited at long intervals by ships that come from South Africa, South America, or even more distant places. One can therefore regard it as a closed community, and there is evidence that epidemics of respiratory disease are introduced from outside.

Records of respiratory symptoms were kept for all the inhabitants over a period of five years. These were then investigated using a hybrid computer, in an attempt to fit them to a model of epidemic spread (see Hammond and Tyrrell, 1971). It was found that a modified Kermack-McKendrick model could be fitted, provided that different parameters were used for each epidemic. On certain occasions it appeared that two simultaneous epidemics had to be postulated.

The symptom patterns and other data suggested that successive epidemics were due to different viruses, and it was therefore quite plausible that the transmission of the virus, and the immunity of the population, varied from epidemic to epidemic. Unfortunately, the study was discontinued before influenza A reached the island, so we have no record of how it spread. Furthermore, it was not possible to collect adequate specimens to identify the viruses circulating or the serological status of the population. However, if someone else could find a sufficiently accessible and cooperative closed community, our experience indicates that it would be possible to gain valuable additional information on the extent to which the values ascribed to the parameters, in order to optimize the fit to the epidemic curve, actually correspond to the features of the real world to which they seem to correspond.

There are examples of influenza epidemics which seem to begin, or to be likely to begin, but which do not in fact "take off". For example, animal influenza viruses with a novel antigenic structure do not usually seem to spread in man, although in the laboratory they behave much like viruses obtained in human epidemics. The recent work of A. S. Beare, at the Common Cold Unit, has shown that many of these viruses infect sero-negative volunteers with considerable difficulty and are shed in small amounts. It seems, therefore, that we should study properties of this sort on "new" viruses. It should be possible to do so without using volunteers; for instance, one might measure the infectious dose and the amount of virus shed in organ cultures of ferret trachea. The stability of the virus on drying could also be measured quite precisely. A combination of such studies might indicate those elements of the transmission parameter (λ) which depend on the virus rather than on the behavior of the human population, and might be used in understanding the occurrence of previous epidemics and the relative potential of future viruses to spread from man to man.

It should also be possible to refine the serological data we already have, in order to estimate the proportion or number of susceptibles in the population. For example, I have used the results of haemagglutination-inhibition tests done in the Sheffield area, supplied to me by Professor C. Potter and Sir Charles Stuart-Harris. From the antibody titers, and the results of challenging volunteers having similar antibody titers at the Common Cold Unit, I have calculated the number of subjects who would be expected to be susceptible. This is not ideal, since the ages of the subjects differ and the challenge virus is a fairly large dose of egg-passaged virus, rather than a naturally-produced aerosol. We do, however, know that resistance detected in this way apparently increases after vaccination, in much the same way as it does under field conditions.

The table shows clearly how the 1968 and following epidemics induced an increased proportion of resistant subjects in the population, and how immunity developed more slowly in the older age groups. It also shows that in 1972 the proportion of subjects who were susceptible to the "new" virus was similar to the proportion susceptible to the 1968 strain in 1968, and that the 1972 virus apparently enhanced resistance to the 1968 strain in the younger age groups, possibly a partial explanation of why the 1968 strain was eliminated. All this information could be used in modelling work on influenza epidemics, perhaps combined with general practitioner records gathered in the same area.

Development of immunity in the population following the appearance of a new strain of influenza virus, by age group

Age	*Percentage susceptible to influenza strain in given year* *A/Hong Kong/68*					*A/Eng/72*	
	1968	*1969*	*1971*	*1972*	*1973*	*1972*	*1973*
0-19	72	56	61	41	24	77	50
20-39	72	54	51	40	28	77	51
40-59	72	61	68	46	46	67	56
60 +	66	65	66	49	49	52	56

It seems to me that the time is now ripe to try to initiate a closer dialogue between those who gather virological information and those who build and evaluate mathematical models. An exchange of ideas and information may trigger off studies which show that, with a little more effort, we can make realistic models of past epidemics and start on the task of predicting the future from the results of laboratory tests.

Reference

Hammond, B.J., and Tyrrell, D.A.J. (1971) A mathematical model of common-cold epidemics on Tristan da Cunha, *J. Hyg., 69,* 423-33.

Session IV: Discussion of presentations by Bailey and Tyrrell

Rapporteur: Pyle

Stuart-Harris suggested that, while developing statistical techniques, we should not forget to consider the properties of the virus and its human host.

Bailey replied that the overall behavior of population dynamics models of the spread of infectious diseases is, to some extent, independent of the detailed characteristics of any particular disease. It depends on how much fine structure (biologically, clinically, etc.) one wants to include. Influenza has special features, and more should be done to incorporate these in the models. He pointed out that the inclusion of a large number of disease parameters, in the interest of realism, can sometimes lead to excessive complications in the modelling process. One should aim to achieve a reasonable balance.

It was pointed out that Tyrrell's method was interesting and might help us to do some modelling without fully understanding what virus we are dealing with. Two contrasting points of view emerged: one was that it is important to understand fully all the biological characteristics of the virus that is being modelled; the other was that one does not actually need to understand the virus fully in order to model the spread of influenza. Clearly, some bridge must be made between these opposing viewpoints. Most participants felt that, in order to maximize reproducibility, rapid serological tests, rapid modifications of the appropriate model to fit the virus, and equally rapid surveillance and control are needed.

Choi pointed out that we must continue to analyze our data carefully, in order to develop retrospective methods that can help explain and forecast severe epidemics.

It was suggested that we should pay particular attention to developing countries if we are to implement such a logical plan of action.

Session V

Herd immunity

Fine

Elveback

Herd immunity (1)

P. E. M. Fine

ABSTRACT

The recognition that the number, proportion, and distribution of the immune individuals in a population are epidemiologically important has given rise to different qualitative and quantitative concepts of "herd immunity". A simple herd immunity threshold, describing the proportion of immunes in a population which leads to reduced incidence, can be derived from simple mass-action theory. However, this omits important factors of total population size and heterogeneity, whose implications are still poorly understood. The herd immunity concept is also related to that of the total (critical) population size necessary to sustain an infection in perpetuity. Although we know this number is approximately 500,000 for measles, we do not know its magnitude for influenza. These concepts may help to explain major changes in influenza ecology, such as the recent appearance of co-circulating viruses.

It was recognized long ago that the number, proportion, and distribution of immune individuals in a population has important epidemiological implications. William Farr noted this as early as 1840, though the term "herd immunity" was apparently not coined until this century, by Greenwood (Wilson, G. S., personal communication; Topley and Wilson, 1923). The concept has rested more on its intuitive reasonableness than on precise definitions, however, and this has led to controversy. Some workers have considered herd immunity a qualitative variable (which a population either has or does not have) whereas others have considered it a quantitative variable (in effect, just another name for the proportion of immunes in a population).

In one sense the herd immunity idea describes an indirect protective effect of immunization, i.e. the immunization of one individual (e.g. by vaccination) removes him as a potential source of infection for those around him, and thus lowers the risk of infection for his unvaccinated neighbors.

In another sense, the herd immunity concept ties in directly with the simple mass-action logic of several models being discussed at this meeting. We return to the basic equation

$$C_{t+1} = C_t \cdot S_t \cdot \lambda_t$$

and recall that the product $S_0\lambda$, called α_0 both in the Russian model and in Spicer's work, is an expression of Macdonald's (1957) basic case reproduction rate (also called the "transmission-to-case ratio", or the "number of effective contacts" of an initial case in an epidemic). In principle, we wish to reduce this below unity to achieve a sort of "herd immunity". If a proportion V are successfully vaccinated, we wish to achieve

$$(1 - V)S_0\lambda < 1$$

which rearranges to

$$V > \frac{S_0\lambda - 1}{S_0\lambda}$$

This is a simple statement of a widely current view of herd immunity. Recalling Spicer's data on influenza, one might suggest a basic reproduction rate $\alpha_0 = S_0\lambda = 5$ (i.e., each case transmits to five others in the early phase of an epidemic). Our simple equation thus says that immunizing more than 80% of a population should reduce the basic case reproduction rate below 1, implying that no epidemic should occur if the infection is introduced under these circumstances.

But it is not that simple. The model assumes a randomly mixing population, and in that sense is dangerously unrealistic. A great deal of experience informs us that infections are maintained in subsets of populations which have special contact patterns, and which are often those subsets that are untouched by vaccination programs. Dr Elveback will discuss this issue of population heterogeneity further, however, so I shall focus on another fallacy in the simple herd immunity concept derived above.

It is unreasonable to expect that the same proportion of immunes would suffice for herd immunity under different population conditions. This is illustrated in Figure 1, which shows the relationship between α_0 (the basic reproduction rate = average number of effective contacts per case) and population size or density. In order to achieve herd immunity, as defined above, we wish to reduce α to below unity, shown by the horizontal interrupted line in the figure. But clearly the effort required to do this will depend on initial α_0 values, and these may vary with different population characteristics. In theory, there could be a constant number of contacts per individual, regardless of population size or density. This situation is represented by line A, and represents the situation where the proportion to be immunized is constant, independent of the population characteristics. In theory it might describe some types of contact infection, perhaps a venereal disease, but certainly not influenza.

FIGURE 1

Relationship between basic case reproduction rate and population size or density

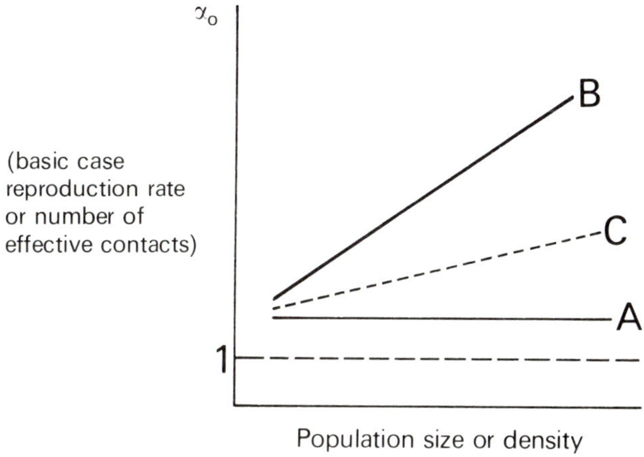

The opposite theoretical extreme is represented by line B, which shows a linear increase in contacts with population size or density. This might be expected in a "pure" airborne infection, in which transmission does not require close proximity to a case. Here, the proportion to be vaccinated in order to reduce α to unity increases with population size or density.

Of course both A and B represent theoretical extremes, and the actual situation is probably represented by a line such as C in the figure. But just where this line might be for any given infection, let alone for influenza, is not known.

In considering herd immunity, we approach the concept of the total population size required to maintain an infectious agent in circulation. This number is sometimes called the "critical population size", and has been most successfully studied with regard to measles (Figure 2). Bartlett (1960), on theoretical grounds, and Black (1966), in studies of island populations, both found that populations of over about 300,000 people were likely to maintain the measles virus in perpetuity, whereas the virus was liable to "fade out" or disappear periodically from smaller populations. Bartlett's theoretical argument was based on a stochastic model. A similar conclusion has been reached by Yorke et al. (1979), but this time based on a deterministic model. These latter authors noted that their deterministic model reproduced the marked seasonal swings of

FIGURE 2

Probability of "fade-out" of measles in relation to total population size

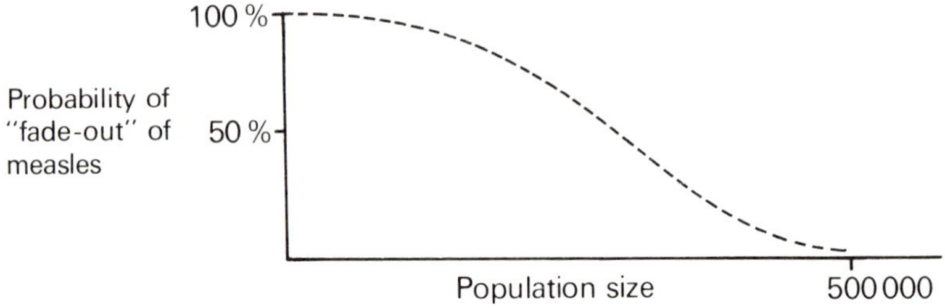

measles. This seasonality is such that only about 0.1% of cases occur during the low month of the year (Figure 3). Thus a population of 500,000, with a birth rate of 20 per 1,000, would expect only ten cases during the seasonal low month. Under this circumstance one might well expect a chance fade-out, the few available cases having, just by chance, no contact with susceptibles.

We might well ask ourselves how relevant such arguments may be for influenza virus patterns and maintenance. The striking seasonality of influenza is obvious. It would appear that only a very small proportion of influenza cases occur during the low-incidence summer months. Does this explain the maintenance or non-maintenance of influenza virus in different populations? I wonder if we may be concentrating too much on epidemic periods, and missing the important implications of those periods when influenza virus is hard to find, or absent. Where does the virus go during the summer? Insofar as public health programs are interested in getting rid of infectious agents, perhaps we could profit by giving greater consideration to how nature appears repeatedly to get rid of influenza viruses.

The issue of how influenza viruses are maintained in populations is one which might profitably be examined with models. Is influenza virus maintained, as is the measles virus, within single large mixing human populations, or does it depend on geographic and population heterogeneity, or "transequatorial swing" (moving from one human population to another, allowing for susceptibles to build up during periods of virus absence), or is the drift-and-shift mechanism essential for virus maintenance? Suppose there were no shift or drift, could influenza virus maintain itself in the human population of today's world? I suspect that this question has more than just rhetorical value, and that it could usefully be investigated using appropriate models.

There is another context in which the concept of critical population size may be relevant to influenza. It was mentioned earlier (in the discussion following Session I) that the pattern of influenza has undergone two major changes in the past century. First, UK records indicate that influenza mortality occurred only irregularly prior to 1890, but that large numbers of influenza deaths have been reported regularly in every year since. Of course, in interpreting such records we must be concerned about diagnostic accuracy and whether this pattern was found elsewhere in the world, but it may well reflect a major change in influenza ecology in the late 19th century.

The second major change occurred in the 1970s, when co-circulation of different shift-type viruses was first recognized. Once again this finding must be examined critically, as it could merely reflect closer surveillance, but most virologists seem to believe that the change is real.

One could argue that these two changes in the epidemiology of influenza are indeed real, and that they reflect increases in the effective size and mixing characteristics of the human host population. The first change occurred in the late 19th century, when ocean transportation by steamships linked the countries of the world closer than ever before. This must have facilitated transmission of infectious agents between previously isolated populations. It may be that, before this time, human populations were too small and isolated to maintain influenza A viruses, and thus those strains which emerged from animal reservoirs exhausted local susceptible groups, only sometimes made it across an ocean, and generally disappeared from the human population within months or years after their appearance. After 1890, communications were sufficient to allow virus strains to circulate throughout the entire human population, crossing oceans and frontiers with ease. In a similar fashion, it may be

FIGURE 3

Seasonal variation in measles incidence

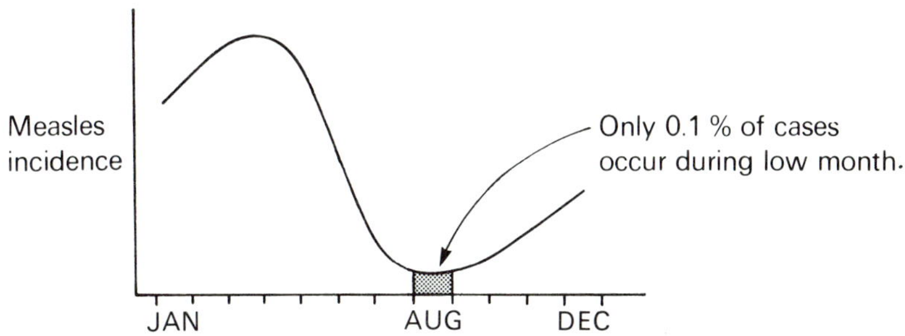

argued that the recent co-circulation of shift-type viruses, despite some degree of cross-protection between them, has been made possible by the combination of a greatly increased world population and the rapid mixing associated with modern transportation, especially by aeroplane. The present world population of almost four billion now acts as a single, non-randomly mixing pool of hosts (with births adding 50 million new susceptibles annually), enough for several viruses together. Granted these thoughts are speculative, but there are times when speculative hypotheses are better than none at all.

References

Bartlett, M. F. (1960) The critical community size for measles in the United States, *J. Roy. Stat. Soc.*, Series A, *123*, 37-44.

Black, F. L. (1966) Measles endemicity in insular populations: Critical community size and its evolutionary implication, *J. Theor. Biol.*, *11*, 207-11.

Farr, W. (1840) *Second report of the Registrar General of England and Wales*, pp. 95-8.

Macdonald, G. (1957) *The epidemiology and control of malaria*, Oxford: Oxford University Press.

Topley, W. W. C. and Wilson, G. S. (1923) The spread of bacterial infection. The problem of herd immunity, *J. Hyg.*, *21*, 243-9.

Yorke, J.A., Nathanson, N., Pianigiani, G., and Martin, J. (1979) Seasonality and the requirements for perpetuation and eradication of viruses in populations, *Amer. J. Epid.*, *109*, 103-23.

Herd immunity (2)

L. R. Elveback

Epidemic potential cannot be measured only in terms of the proportion of the population who are immune, or in terms of the number of susceptibles alone. It is essential to consider the clustering of the susceptibles (Fox et al., 1971; Fox and Elveback, 1975).

Clustering may be geographic, as in the centers of cities in the USA, where levels of immunity tend to be very low among people who are not covered by health services. Sometimes this is because they do not speak English, and are therefore not aware of the medical services that are available. For example, sending out notices in English, with the telephone bill, to a cluster of Spanish-speaking people has been shown to be of very little help. It is expensive and time-consuming to achieve adequate levels of immunization in such clusters, but it may be worthwhile as they help to support epidemics.

In West Africa, it is the infants who are the most susceptible to measles. Clustering of infants occurs as a result of mothers carrying their babies to the market-place. Consequently, measles continues to attack these infants despite their very high levels of immunity (Millar, 1969; Millar and Foege, 1969).

Clusters may be social, rather than geographic. For example the Abakalike, in eastern Nigeria, refused vaccination on religious grounds. Although they were dispersed throughout the community, they maintained frequent contact with each other and sustained endemic smallpox (Foege, personal communication).

There is still another problem. Even with random mixing and a high level of immunity in all groups of the population, the concept of herd immunity breaks down with airborne spread. Transmission of the virus can occur without direct person-to-person contact, as has been demonstrated by recent outbreaks on an aeroplane and on a ship. Thus "exposure" and "contact" are not the same.

It is apparent that, if the term "herd immunity" is to have any useful interpretation, it must be both limited and complex.

References

Fox, J. P., Elveback, L, Scott W., Gatewood, L., and Ackerman, E. (1971) Herd immunity: basic concept and relevance to public health immunization practices, *Amer. J. Epid.*, *94*, 179-89.

Fox, J.P., and Elveback, L.R. (1975) Herd immunity–changing concepts, in: *Viral Immunology and Immunopathology*, Chapter 16, London and New York: Academic Press.

Millar, J.D. (1969) "Measles control in Africa: A practical and theoretical epidemiologic challenge" (Unpublished paper, presented at the annual meeting of the American Public Health Association, Philadelphia, November 1969).

Millar, J.D., and Foege, W.H. (1969) Status of eradication of smallpox (and control of measles) in West and Central Africa, *J. infect. Dis.*, *120*, 725-32.

Session V: Discussion of presentations by Fine and Elveback

Rapporteur: Bailey

It was first pointed out that the Tristan da Cunha experience with the common cold showed, by fitting curves to actual data, that epidemics occurred in conditions well above the relevant threshold, and herd immunity worked better than expected. However, one member of the group wondered how much one could really tell about herd immunity if large numbers of different viruses were involved. Perhaps there was no immunity to new viruses.

It was suggested that what happened in practice was a kind of average over several different parallel outbreaks, but the implications of this for herd immunity were unclear.

Generally speaking, modelling could help to examine different hypotheses and test them. In particular, one could ask why fade-out occurred or, alternatively, why it did not occur. To investigate this problem of extinction necessitated the use of stochastic models, but it should not be forgotten that better data might be required for satisfactory results. Good data collection might be difficult. One aspect of this was that influenza virus-induced infections might still be occurring in relatively quiescent periods, but these would not necessarily be directly revealed by the ordinary reports from general practitioners. In the context of insect pests such as aphids, it was not the level of winter kill that mattered, since a few individuals would always survive. It was the rate of increase in the spring that was really important. Similar considerations might apply to the rapid spread of influenza under favorable conditions following a period of quiescence.

The differences between different viral infections in humans were especially emphasized. In measles, for example, there is low lethality and a state of relative equilibrium *vis-à-vis* the human host. But with influenza strong immunity is liable to develop to individual strains, and the virus has to keep changing its structure in order to survive. This is a consequence of disobeying the rule: "never kill your host if you want to survive", and may explain the disappearance of some strains and the emergence of new ones.

It was noted, however, that influenza B virus shows only very slow antigenic changes, while strains of influenza A virus exhibit more rapid modifications. In addition, some new variants might reinforce immunity to older ones. Of course, genetic changes occur in all organisms. It is relevant to ask how much we need to assume about such changes, in order to explain observed phenomena. Because of its adaptability, it might be said that influenza is more successful than measles in maintaining itself.

The importance of different population subgroups, especially in regard to vaccination strategies, was also stressed. Children should be given special attention. However, one member of the group pointed out that the routine compulsory vaccination of children in Japan had little effect on the course of influenza epidemics.

There was some speculation about what really happened in the UK during periods of low incidence, and it was suggested that inter-epidemic periods might require a different kind of modelling; with polio, for example, the infection might be kept going during such periods by means of isolated infections. However, a counter-suggestion was made that it may not be essential to adopt structurally different models, but that more insight and understanding might be obtained by retaining the same underlying model, and possibly changing some of the parameters in accordance with changes in external conditions.

There was further discussion of the phenomenon of herd immunity as such. This is presumably a function of the number of susceptibles and the contact rate, which is itself a parameter that varies during the year. More information is needed on the kind of variation that actually occurs, with respect to annual changes, weather conditions, school entrances, etc., taking into account both the total population and identifiable sub-populations. The USSR model, as applied, assumes a constant basic infection rate. This assumption might be valid over periods of a few weeks, but perhaps not over months.

The importance of distinguishing cases of infection, as opposed to disease, was accepted, but it was considered that this did not raise any new fundamental issues. The use of appropriate parameters in existing models could take care of the distinction. In any case it was of more fundamental importance to model infection, rather than disease.

There was discussion of how much virological, serological, and immunological detail should be included in models. Good data are available from some communities, and it is desirable to follow the populations over long periods of time, e.g. ten years. In particular, measurements of the relative proportions of those who are serologically positive or negative should be made after any given epidemic is over.

Problems of vaccination were then reviewed. It was pointed out that, in one country where mass vaccination against polio had protected most people, a religious community that remained unprotected showed an appreciable incidence. It was emphasized that, while a killed vaccine (e.g. Salk) could achieve immunity only for vaccinated individuals, an attenuated live vaccine (e.g. Sabin) could spread immunity to many other susceptible individuals in the community.

As regards influenza control, it was pointed out that an assessment should be made of relative costs and benefits. For example, the production of a new vaccine to carry out a public health intervention might be very expensive, while the consequences of an uncontrolled outbreak might be small. There might also be adverse reactions to the vaccine. In addition, account should be taken of the fact that some influenza strains affect only children, while others affect many older people. Perhaps too much attention has been given to antigenic differences, whereas more emphasis should be laid on achieving immunity to actual disease.

It was reiterated that experience in the USSR showed that relatively simple modelling could account for the observed phenomena in terms of the occurrence and spread of influenza over quite widely separated population centers. These insights could undoubtedly be developed in order to find a wide range of applications elsewhere.

Finally, it was suggested that the original concepts and definitions involved in "herd immunity" should now be replaced by the more precise quantitative notions that had been discussed and that were capable of describing and explaining a broad spectrum of serological and epidemiological phenomena. So far as influenza is concerned, effective control might be nearer than we realize, especially in view of the rapid fade-out which occurs soon after the appearance of many new viral strains.

Abstract of discussion

1. In measles there is low lethality and relative equilibrium *vis-à-vis* the human host, whereas in influenza the occurrence of strong immunity in humans to individual strains implies that the virus has to change its structure in order to survive.

2. Questions were raised as to how much virological, serological, and immunological detail should be included in a quantitative model.

3. As some strains, like influenza B, show only slow antigenic changes, it is important to ask how much change is required in relation to immunity in order to explain the observed phenomena.

4. It is important to distinguish infections from cases of disease. The process of infection is epidemiologically more fundamental, its occurrence being represented in a model by an appropriate parameter.

5. Different population subgroups should be distinguished, particularly children and especially in relation to vaccination strategies.

6. Models could help to examine and test different hypotheses. In particular, probabilistic models are required to investigate problems of fade-out and extinction.

7. The influenza modelling done in the USSR is capable of explaining the dynamic phenomena of spatial spread over large geographic areas. It could probably be developed for even wider applications elsewhere.

8. Questions were raised as to the precise nature of what happens to the influenza virus during periods of very low disease incidence. Could the same underlying population model be used, possibly with changes in the parameters reflecting changes in external conditions?

9. Attention was drawn to the importance of cost-benefit studies in relation to influenza control, contrasting for example the costs of producing a new vaccine and of possible adverse reactions with the benefits of preventing the expected consequences of an uncontrolled outbreak.

10. It was proposed that the concept of "herd immunity" should be discarded and replaced by more modern ideas that are better capable of describing and explaining the wide spectrum of observed serological and epidemiological phenomena.

SESSION VI

Models of geographic spread

Haggett

Pyle

Choi

Building geographic components into epidemiological models

P. Haggett

ABSTRACT

A study of measles in Iceland showed it to have an intricate pattern of geographic spread. Comparison of successive epidemics confirmed the presence of weak but detectable regularities, which can be reproduced in spatial models and which permit some hope that epidemiological models with reasonable forecasting capability can be built.

Three areas of potential relevance to influenza modelling are:

(1) the identification of pathways of viral spread,

(2) the extension of both time-series and epidemiological models by adding spatial components, and

(3) the construction of risk maps and early-warning systems.

Extension of such work to influenza is under way.

While the world's population has doubled over the last generation, its spatial mobility has increased by a factor of perhaps 200. During the 1980s we can expect a total population approaching five billion, and an annual passenger flow of over a billion by air travel alone. The slowly-changing geographic distribution of susceptibles, and the rapidly-changing patterns of interaction between different areas, both need to be considered in designing epidemiological models for use on a large geographic scale.

I shall summarize the work of a small group of geographers and statisticians in England, who are involved in this task. The group consists of Dr A.D. Cliff (Cambridge University), Dr J.K. Ord (Warwick University), and myself, assisted by postgraduate students, notably some who are reading for the diploma in mathematical statistics under Professor D. G. Kendall, at Cambridge University. The work published so far, and summarized in Cliff and Haggett (1980) and Cliff et al. (1981), is concerned with measles, an infectious disease with a very simple transmission pattern, located in a single isolated geographic area, namely Iceland (Figure 1). Extension to epidemiological models of a

FIGURE 1

The Bartlett model of virus transmissions between geographically separate communities of different sizes. For measles, Iceland forms a type B community.

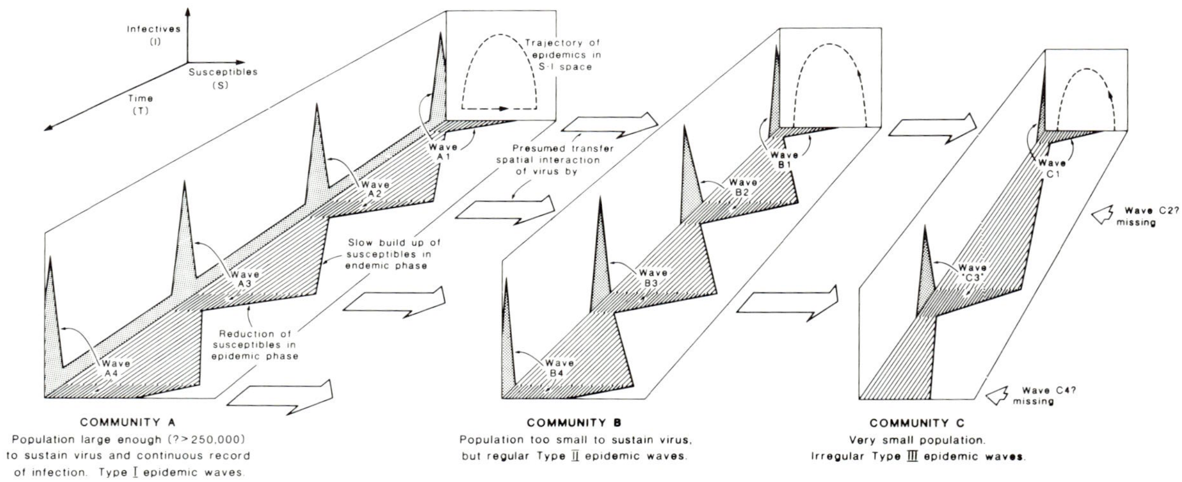

more complex viral disease such as influenza, and to larger and more complex geographic areas, imposes much more stringent requirements. Our group has begun a study of influenza epidemics in Iceland, but there are no substantive findings to report yet. The comments which follow are therefore largely confined to our experience with measles.

Three aspects of the group's work which may be of most relevance to epidemiological modelling are: (1) the identification of pathways of viral spread, (2) the addition of spatial components to models of epidemics, and (3) the constuction of risk maps. Each is discussed in turn.

1. Identification of pathways of viral spread

A partial picture of the ways in which viruses spread through a population with a particular geographic distribution can sometimes be constructed from the published records of public health authorities. Three methods which the team have used are described.

(a) Provenance of index cases using physicians' records

Published records of infectious diseases in Iceland stretch back in considerable detail to the 1890s. Accompanying the annual reports by the central public health authority are digests of written reports by local physicians, describing outbreaks within their area and, for some diseases, the movements of those infected individuals (the index cases) who first brought the infection into a local area. Plotting the provenance of index cases for 17 measles epidemics allowed us to study the spread pattern of an individual epidemic (Figure 2). By accumulating results from successive outbreaks, we were able to plot the general distribution of pathways of viral spread, their seasonal variations (Figure 3), and changes over time as transport linkages changed. Knowledge of the actual movement of index cases, from physicians' observations, provided a useful check on any presumed spread of infectives, as in the mass-action models, and allowed comparison with passenger flows between local areas.

(b) Pathways inferred from spatial autocorrelation studies

When direct evidence of spread is lacking, we have to fall back on the indirect evidence of records giving only the place and time of onset. While we may be tempted to add vectors to a map of onset dates, in order to indicate the presumed pathways of viral spread, this is a rather subjective process, since usually there are many different trajectories over which infection may be carried. Spatial autocorrelation studies can be used

FIGURE 2a

Reported pathways of measles virus spread for the fifth of the 17 measles epidemics that have occurred in Iceland since the 1890s

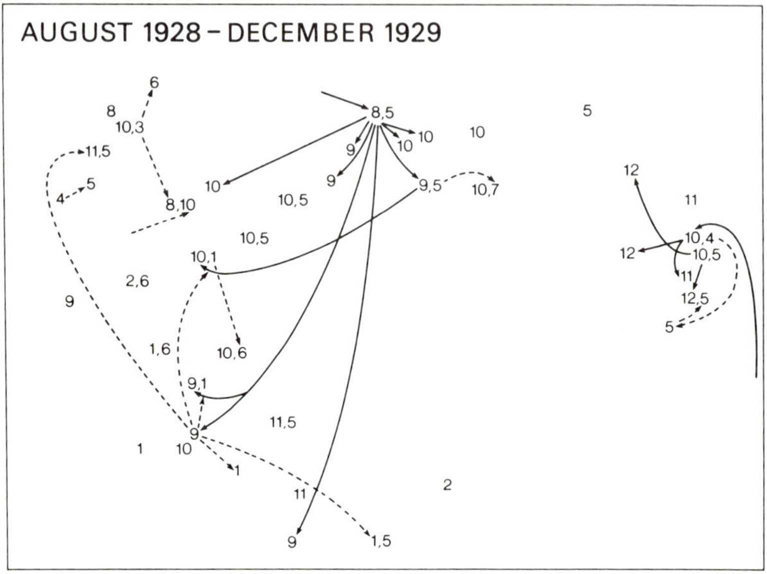

Arrows link the origins and destinations of infected individuals, according to physicians' reports, but do not attempt to show their actual routes. The solid lines refer to 1928, the broken lines to 1929. The numbers refer to months within those years. From Cliff et al., 1981.

to differentiate between alternative hypothetical pathways and to identify the most probable pattern of spread. An application of this method to measles outbreaks is described in Haggett (1976) and Cliff et al. (1981).

(c) Regional comparison of epidemic velocities

We tried to find the most appropriate way to measure accurately the progress of an epidemic when treated as a wave phenomenon (Cliff and Haggett, 1982). We showed that, for 13 major measles outbreaks in Iceland between 1916 and 1974, the wave velocities in urban and rural populations tended to converge, as a result of their slowing down in the former and accelerating in the latter. These findings are consistent with the hypothesis that improved communications are allowing a speeding-up of viral transmission *between* populations, but a slowing-down *within* populations (although whether this is due to improved preventive measures, such as vaccination levels, is unclear). We are now conducting similar studies on the speed of spread of influenza waves.

FIGURE 2b

Measles epidemic of August 1928–December 1929

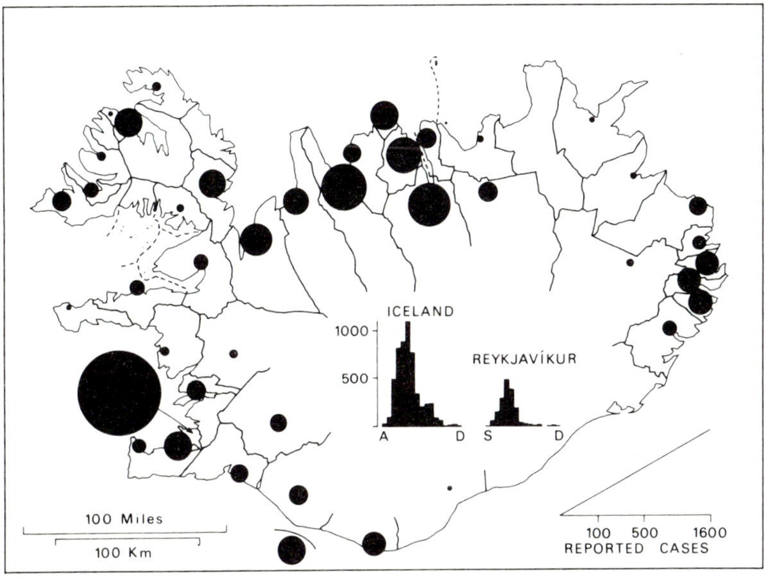

The areas of the circles are proportional to the total number of measles cases reported in each medical district during the epidemic. The scale for the circles is given in the lower right-hand corner. The histograms give the number of reported cases by month for Iceland and Reykjavik (A = August 1928, S = September 1928, D = December 1929). From Cliff et al., 1981.

Spatial components in epidemiological models

The group's work on modelling measles epidemics in Iceland involved a wide range of methods (see table). The following comments summarize our experience (Cliff et al., 1981):

1. No "Rosetta stone" model which gives reasonable projections of epidemic recurrences and epidemic size was found. Generally, if a model is devised which will forecast recurrences acceptably, it overestimates epidemic size. This is because, in order to forecast recurrences, the model must be sensitive to changes signalling the approach of an epidemic, with the result that it "overshoots" when the epidemic is in progress.

2. Models which are based only on the size of the infective population in previous time-periods consistently fail to detect the approach of an epidemic. They do, however, provide reasonable estimates of the number of cases reported, but tend to run in arrears.

3. Models with parameters fixed through time tend to smooth out the highs and lows of an epidemic, because they are unable to adapt to the changes between the build-up and fade-out phases. Time-varying parameter models are better at avoiding this problem.

4. Epidemic recurrences can be forecast only by incorporating into the model information on the size of the susceptible population and/or

FIGURE 3

Pathways of viral spread as shown by movements of index cases in measles epidemics (1896-1975), by month of occurrence. The role of the capital city Reykjavik (R) as a source of infection, and the greater number of contacts in early summer, are shown.

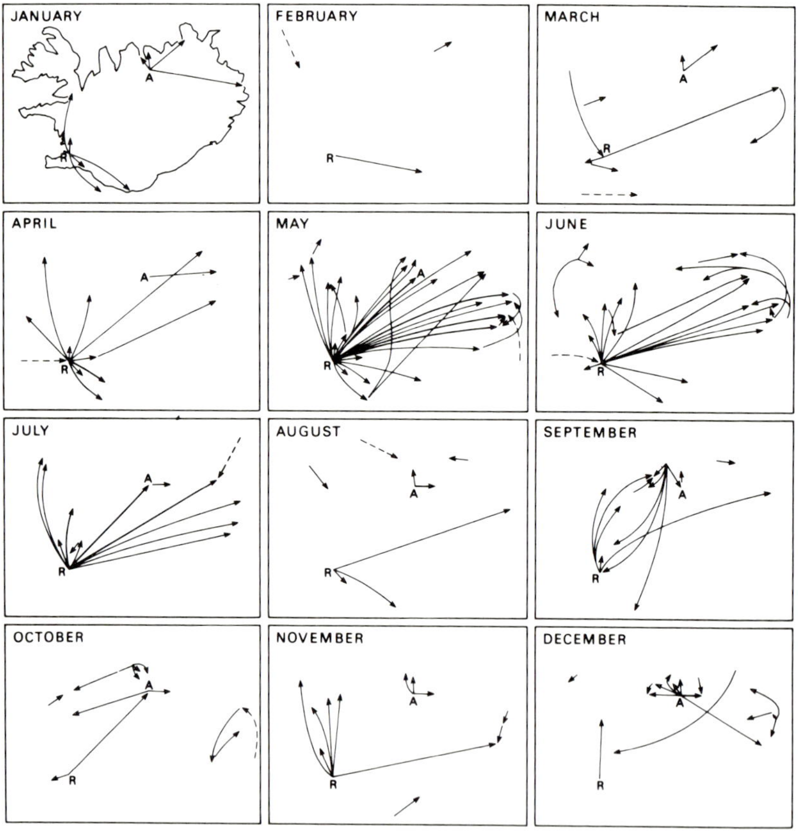

From Cliff et al., 1981.

Experience of the use of epidemic models in the Iceland measles survey

Models used

- Time-series models
  - Autoregressive models AR (1)
    - With fixed parameters

      One-period[a] lag effect; consistently miss epidemic starts; reasonable estimates of epidemic size.
    - With time-varying parameters (Kalman)

      Initial one-period[a] lag effect; able to adapt to changing phase characteristics; over-estimates epidemic size.
  - Generalized linear integrated models (GLIM)

    Use of major settlement as epidemic lead indicator produces good estimates of epidemic starts in other medical districts in the surrounding region. Poor estimates of epidemic size.
- Epidemiological models
  - Hamer-Soper models

    Good ability to forecast epidemic recurrences some years ahead. Average to poor on estimates of epidemic size.
  - Chain-binomial models

    Initial one-period[a] lag effect; able to lock onto course of epidemic; reasonable estimates of epidemic size. Little improvement by adopting a time-varying parameter. Results for multi-area case similar to GLIM.

[a] Period = reporting period. This was one month, but could be reduced to one week or less with an appropriate data-collecting system.
From Cliff et al., 1981.

properly identifying the lead-lag structure among medical districts for disease transmission. Incorporation of information on spatial interaction markedly improves our ability to forecast recurrences in lagging areas. Information on the number of susceptibles in a population also serves to prime a model to the possibility of a recurrence, as is made clear by the various threshold theorems. Models based on susceptible populations, but which are single- rather than multi-regional, tend to miss the start of an epidemic but rapidly lock on to its course thereafter. Models which are dominated by information on spatial transmission, at the expense of information on the number of susceptibles in the population in the reference region, produce estimates of epidemic size which reflect the course of the epidemic in the triggering regions, rather than in the reference region.

5. Process models serve to strengthen the time-series models, and are better for forecasting.

The above comments emphasize the fact that naive models produce poor results. However, the table indicates the gains to be made for each extra element of complexity added to our models, namely:

1. Time-varying parameters to handle the non-stationary nature of within-epidemic structure, particularly the fundamentally different nature of the build-up and fade-out phases of an epidemic.

2. Spatial lead-lag information, to improve our ability to forecast epidemic recurrences.

3. Incorporation of an estimate of the number of susceptibles in a population, to improve estimates of epidemic size and likely recurrence intervals.

It is important to be able to identify the gains due to increasing model complexity, since it is all too easy to specify sophisticated models which often achieve little more than simple trend predictors, yet are much harder to use.

Risk maps and spatial early-warning systems

Study of the Icelandic records suggests that the geographic spread of epidemics is neither deterministic and well-behaved, nor wholly chaotic and random. Given the present state of knowledge, it seems improbable that any of the epidemic models with which we have experience will precisely forecast the exact arrival time, intensity, and eventual size of a measles wave in any area. But it is possible to make better estimates of the *likelihood* of waves of a given character occurring at particular times and places. (A useful analogy may be made with the life-tables drawn up by actuaries. These do not predict the life-span of a single individual, but rather the life-expectancy based on the study of a population's cohorts.)

Current work in Iceland on the prediction of measles epidemics includes producing risk maps which can be updated at weekly intervals. For an area not currently reporting the disease, the risk of an outbreak in the next time-period is seen as a function of three major factors:

1. The *spatial vulnerability* of an area, in terms of its nearness to already infected areas. Here "nearness" is measured, not in terms of distance, but as a function of the flow of individuals between the two areas. While this may sometimes be directly recorded from traffic and passenger records, more commonly it has to be estimated from standard spatial interaction models (Haggett et al., 1977). Where more than one area is infected, the different source areas are integrated to give a general measure of spatial vulnerability.

2. The *epidemiological vulnerability* of an area, in terms of its susceptible population. This may sometimes be estimated from serological sampling, but more usually has to be reconstructed from the age structure of the population, the previous pattern of infections, and the level of immunization achieved by past vaccination programs.

3. The *temporal vulnerability* of the area, in terms of general seasonal factors plus the expected frequency of any climatic triggers (e.g. sudden temperature changes) that might predispose to complications arising from an initial infection. In the case of influenza, an antigenic shift would be a critical factor under this heading.

It is easier to identify the factors entering into any forecast of risk than to estimate the specific weights to be attached to each factor. Each factor requires separate estimating equations and, as in any forecasts, there is a need to balance the formal projection system by the experience of the public health official issuing the forecast for any area.

The practical value of a forecast as an early-warning device depends on the lead-time it provides in relation to the time needed to prepare counter-measures. The post-war measles epidemics in Iceland show a distinct regional pattern (Figure 4), with lags of several months between first reports of outbreaks in the capital city and in progressively more remote rural areas. Careful study of the geography of other infectious diseases might allow similar atlases of lead-lag times to be built up, both at the international level and within individual countries. Where such lags occur from the center to the periphery, are reasonably stable

FIGURE 4

Average lag times, in months, between the start of a measles epidemic and the arrival of the first reported case in various districts

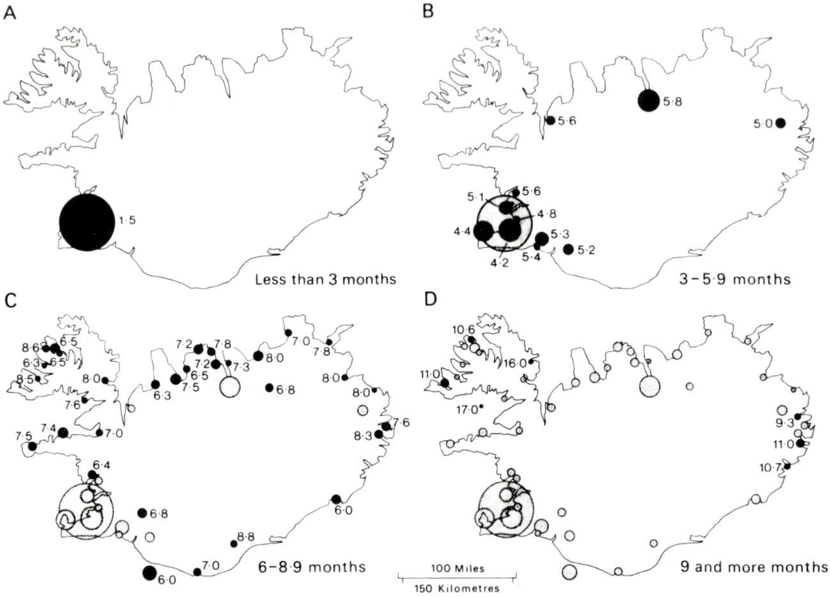

From Cliff and Haggett, 1979.

from one outbreak to another, and are long in relation to the lead-time needed for large-scale vaccine production, there are grounds for believing that an early-warning system would be useful.

References

Cliff, A. D., and Haggett, P. (1980) Geographical aspects of epidemic diffusion in closed communities, in Wrigley, N., ed., *Statistical applications in the spatial sciences,* London: Prior/Methuen, 5-44.

Cliff, A. D., and Haggett, P. (1981) Measuring the velocity of epidemic waves, *Int. J. Epid., 11,* 82-9.

Cliff, A. D., Haggett, P., Ord, J. K., and Versey, G. R. (1981) *Spatial diffusion: an historical geography of epidemics in an island community,* Cambridge: Cambridge University Press.

Haggett, P. (1976) Hybridizing alternative models of an epidemic diffusion process, *Economic Geography, 52,* 136-46.

Haggett, P., Cliff, A. D., and Frey, A. E. (1977) *Locational analysis in human geography,* 2nd ed., London: Edward Arnold.

Some observations on the geography of influenza diffusion

G. F. Pyle

ABSTRACT

An historical survey of the influenza literature indicated that different viral strains show variable patterns and rates of spatial diffusion. A more specific geographic analysis of the spread of influenza during the late 1960s showed that the resurgence of H_2N_2 during the winter of 1967-68 had a dampening effect on the diffusion of H_3N_2 during the following season. During both periods, influenza diffusion "fields" formed as early source areas of outbreaks.

I shall present some preliminary findings on the geographic aspects of influenza diffusion. In order to develop a method that might help to explain the diffusion of influenza, and perhaps to forecast future paths of spread, a long historical view was taken, including the examination of narrative historical accounts from the 1500s up to and including the 1918-19 pandemic. Geographic aspects of influenza after the discovery of the virus, in 1933, were then examined from the late 1930s up to the late 1960s. Preliminary studies are in progress for the late 1970s and early 1980s.

There is a certain conventional wisdom about the geographic spread of influenza. It includes a "Eurocentric" view that influenza epidemics always start somewhere else, probably in China or Central Asia. It also states that influenza spreads geographically in waves, from points of origin outward, with little or no respect for transportation systems. Through archival research it was possible to reconstruct epidemics of the 1500s, 1600s, 1700s, and 1800s. These generalized accounts indicate that there may in fact have been a rather wave-like progression of many epidemics through Europe, but they did not all necessarily originate in Central Asia. The epidemic of 1580 is particularly well documented, and there is evidence from historical accounts indicating that it spread from Russia through Europe and into England. Information on epidemics in the 1700s is much better than earlier accounts. In some instances, for example in 1782, it appears that influenza may have spread from North America to Europe. Accounts in the early 1800s indicate some diffusion of influenza from South America to Europe.

In general, an examination of several early epidemics indicates that influenza does not always start in the same places within Europe and England, but that it can spread in regular, wave-like paths once the virus has been seeded. Spring seeding can be identified in some historical accounts, and there is some indication that less severe forms of influenza may seed in certain geographic locations in the spring and then diffuse outward from adjacent places during the following autumn. Evidence suggests that this occurred in the epidemic of 1889-92. A geographic analysis of the major pandemic of 1918-19 indicates some form of spring activity during 1918 in North America, although the origins of the epidemics are not well known because of its extreme severity and rapid spread through various parts of the world from 1918 to 1920.

By the 1920s the cyclical nature of influenza was well known, as a result of improvements in statistical measuring techniques. Knowledge of the temporal and spatial distribution of influenza epidemics was greatly enhanced with the discovery of the virus, in 1933. Examination of an epidemic in the USA prior to that discovery, in 1928-29, also suggests some evidence of seeding, with the diffusion of influenza outwards from central parts of the country to western and then eastern locations. Thus, even prior to the discovery of the virus, there is some indication of influenza endemicity within North America, as well as of ecological conditions that give rise to alterations in viruses and subsequent "new" epidemics.

Two major outbreaks in the 1940s were analyzed geographically. The first was an epidemic of what was then termed "influenza A", during the winter of 1943-44. During that particular season there is additional evidence of early outbreaks in the Mississippi delta and interior areas of the USA, with subsequent diffusion to coastal locations. Another virus, then presumed to be different from the one mentioned above (now designated as H_1N_1), was reported during the 1947-48 influenza season within the USA. It was much less virulent than the 1943-44 virus, suggesting that they were different strains, but its geographic diffusion pattern was somewhat similar to the earlier virus although much less intense.

A geographic analysis of the diffusion of H_2N_2 within the USA demonstrated a clearly different pattern from the viruses of the 1940s. It appears initially to have entered the country along both the east and west coasts, and to have diffused inland. However, there is strong evidence of early outbreaks at several interior locations, as well as in the Mississippi delta area and Texas with diffusion toward more inland parts of the country. Some parts of the USA which demonstrated the earliest broad regional outbreaks were not necessarily the more densely populated. However, influenza quickly spread to major centers of population.

The introduction of the Hong Kong (H_3N_2) strain into the USA demonstrated a rather enigmatic pattern. Part of the diffusion of that virus, which is difficult to explain, is due to a flare-up of H_2N_2 during the 1967-68 influenza season. Cases due to a presumed endemic virus reached epidemic proportions. Furthermore, the introduction of H_3N_2 into the population, perhaps as early as the spring of 1968, resulted in a "double peaking", in which the 1968-69 influenza season was also of epidemic proportions. Some researchers have pointed out that the two strains are sufficiently related for the higher-than-expected rates during the 1967-68 season to have had a dampening effect on the diffusion of H_3N_2 throughout the USA the following winter. In fact, county data from the National Center for Health Statistics show that many parts of the USA did have higher peaks during the 1967-68 season than the following winter, as shown in Figure 1.

Given the presumed endemic nature of the prevailing viral strain, it was not surprising to find regional clusters of outbreaks within the USA during the late summer and early autumn of 1967. Figures 2 and 3 show "primary" and "secondary" regional clusters of H_2N_2 outbreaks during that time period. The thick arrows indicate the major diffusion pathways. When the primary and secondary outbreaks are combined, as shown in Figure 4, influenza diffusion "fields" can be identified for most of the USA during the beginning of the 1967-68 epidemic. The two strongest indicators of such movement proved to be geographic adjacency to core areas and distance from epicenters of outbreaks. As has been observed in the influenza literature, major transportation routes were not as important as direct spatial diffusion.

The outbreak of H_3N_2 was indeed dampened by the rapid influenza diffusion during the previous season. Figures 5 and 6 give some indication of primary and secondary outbreaks of influenza during the late summer and autumn of 1968. A different virus, but apparently with some similar characteristics to H_2N_2, had also shown epidemic seeding in the form of regional clusters. Many, but certainly not all, of those parts of the USA which experienced the strongest early outbreaks during the 1967-68 season surprisingly showed less severity and slower reporting during the 1968-69 season. Still, a "new" virus had entered the country, and by the late autumn of 1968 influenza diffusion fields had covered most of it (see Figure 7).

While there is, without doubt, a certain amount of randomness both within the data sets used and the actual seeding of two different influenza viruses during epidemic periods, the disease did not spread in large waves. In addition, co-mingling of viruses was clearly taking place at that

FIGURE 1

Regions with highest reporting during epidemics: 1967-68 (H_2N_2) and 1968-69 (H_3N_2)

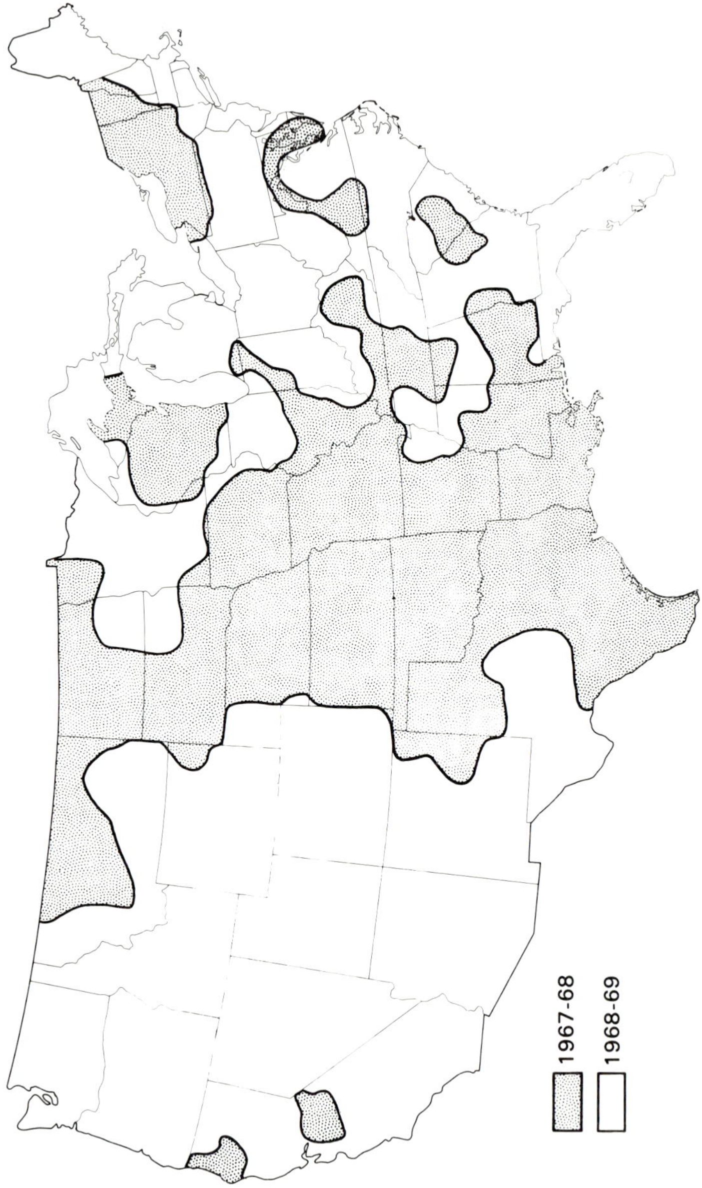

FIGURE 2
Core areas and diffusion pathways for primary outbreaks of influenza during the beginning of the 1967-68 season

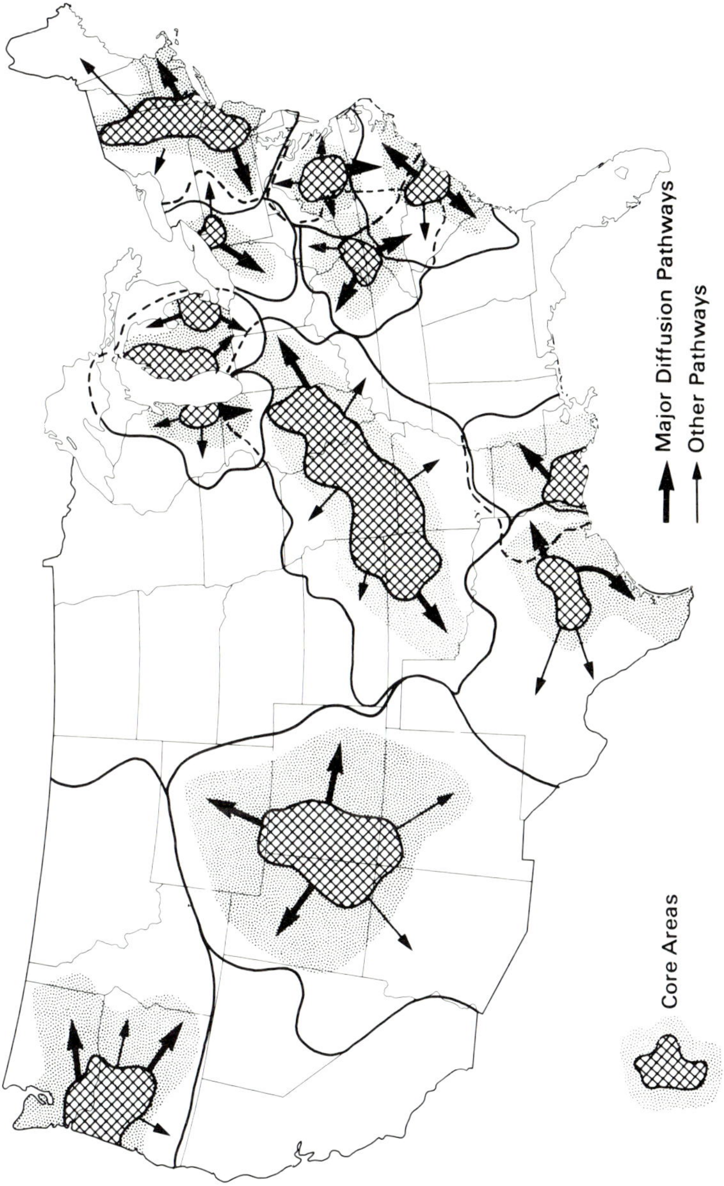

FIGURE 3

Core areas and diffusion pathways for secondary outbreaks of influenza, 1967-68

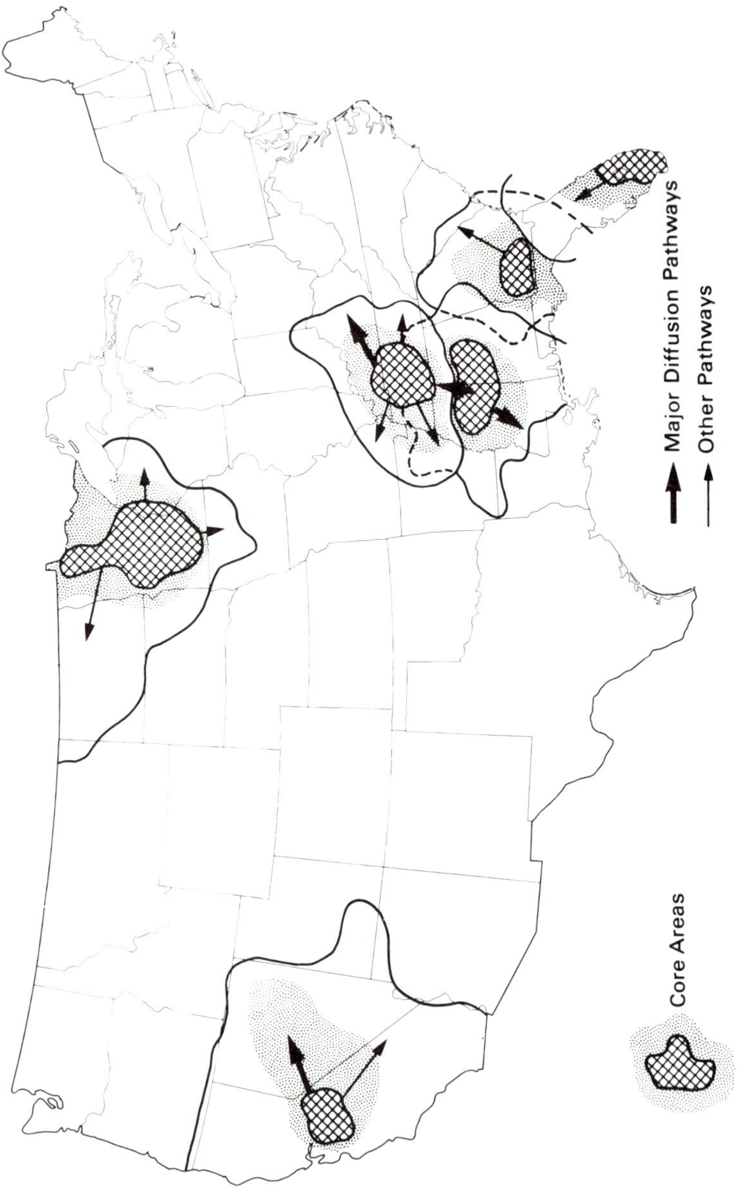

FIGURE 4

Influenza "fields" during the beginning of the 1967-68 epidemic

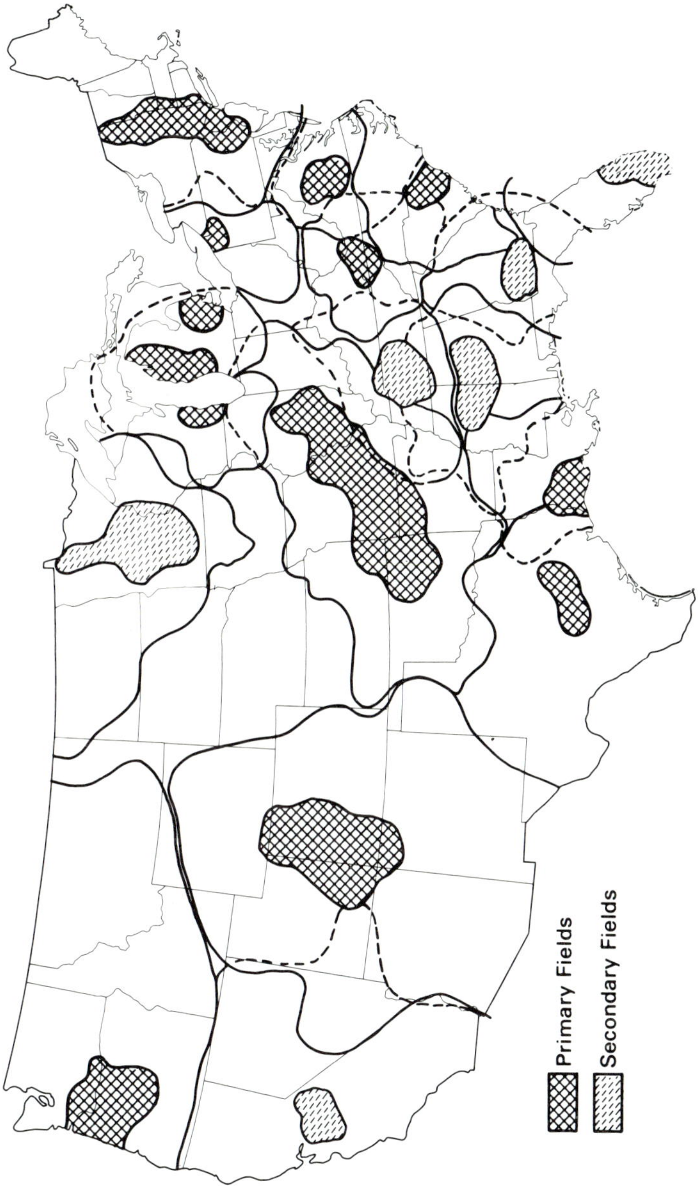

FIGURE 5

Core areas and diffusion pathways for primary outbreaks of influenza during the beginning of the 1968-69 season

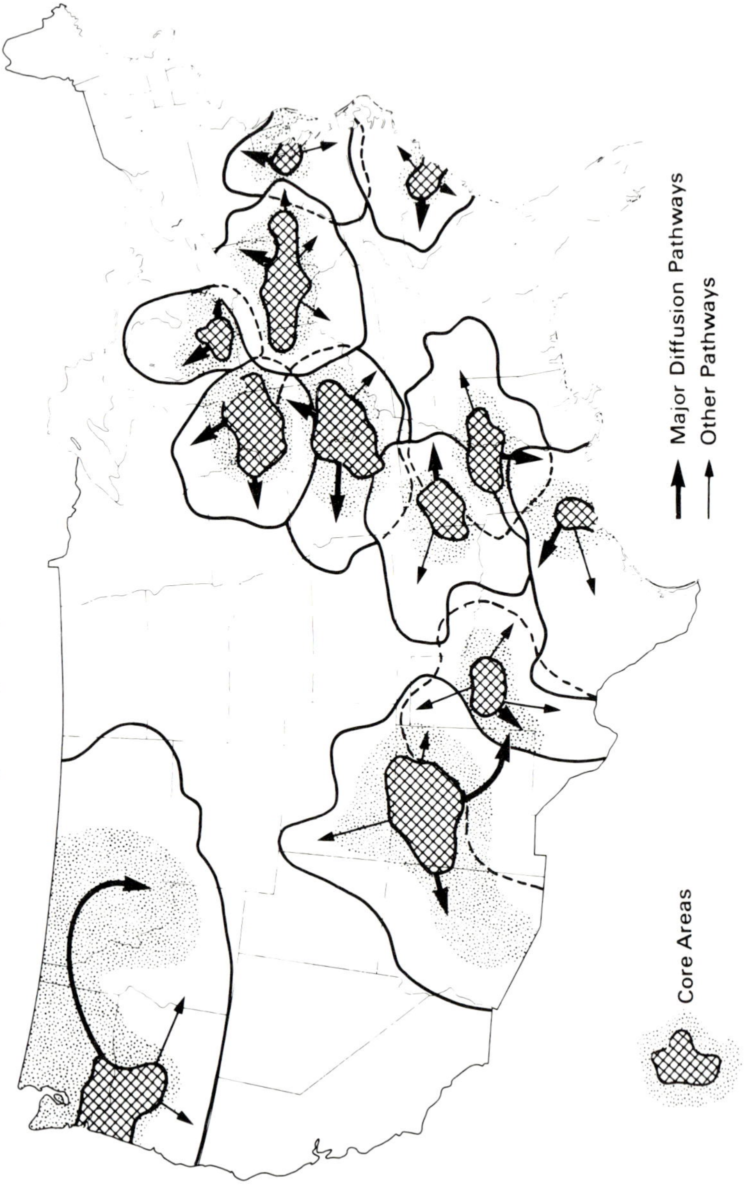

FIGURE 6

Core areas and diffusion pathways for secondary outbreaks of influenza, 1968-69

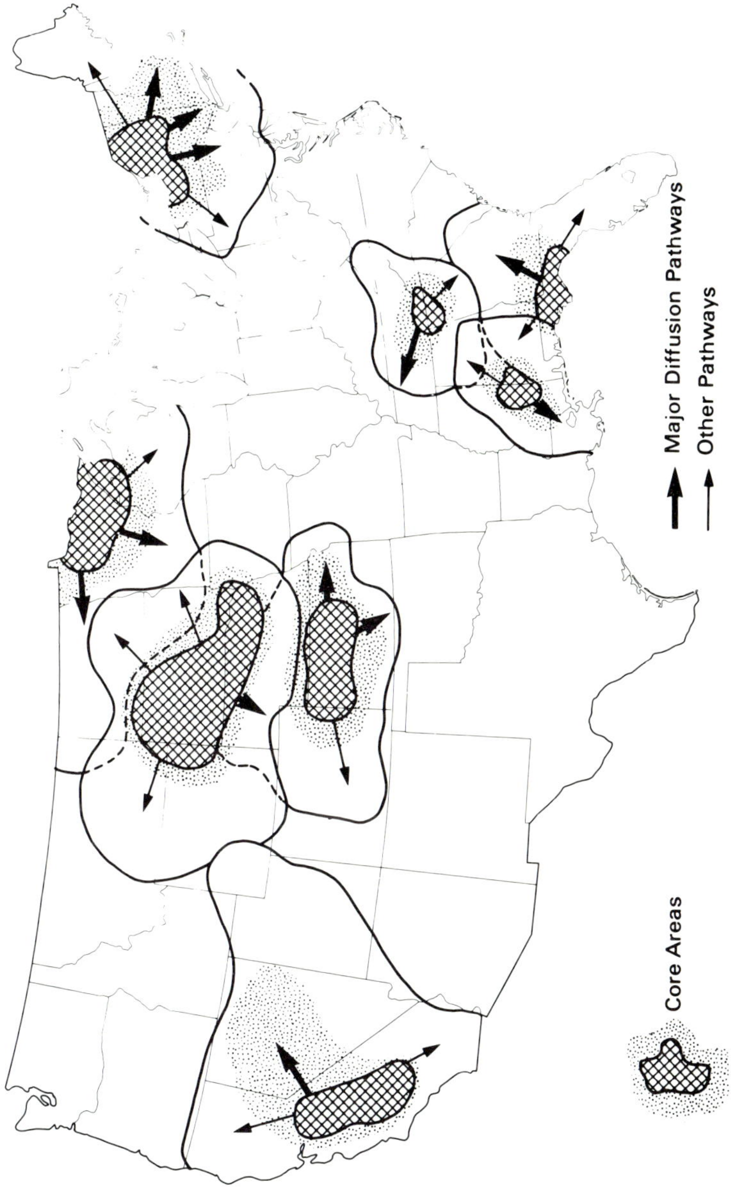

FIGURE 7

Influenza "fields" during the beginning of the 1968-69 epidemic

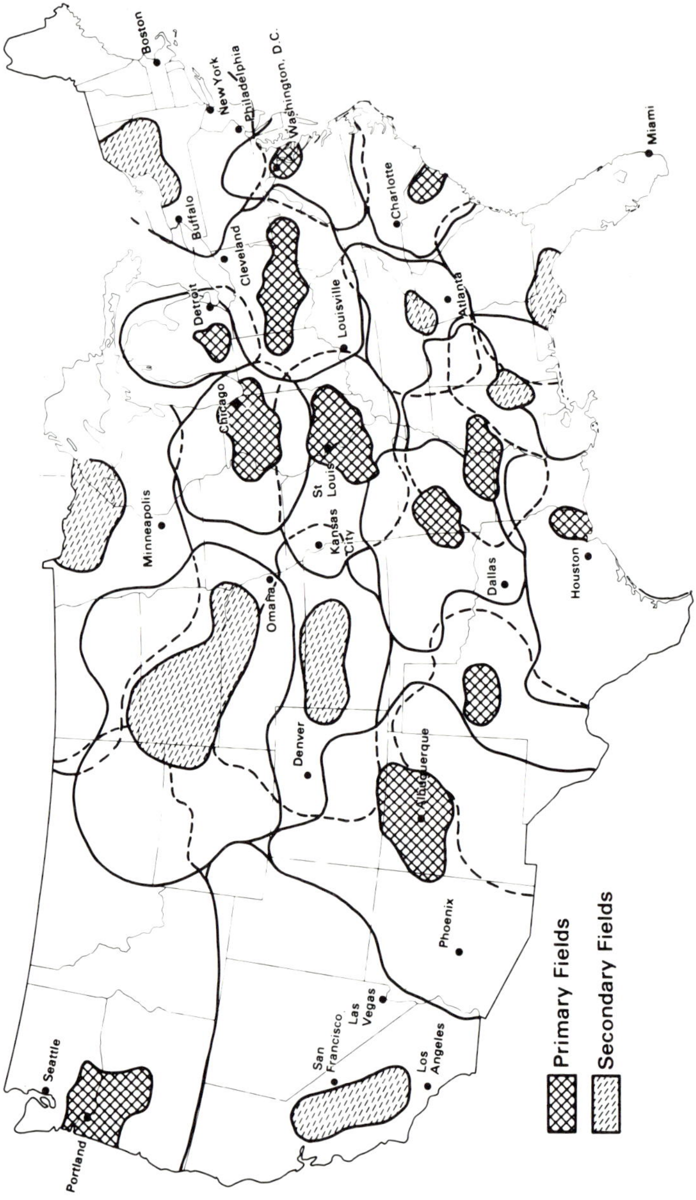

time. With respect to *when* and *where* the seeding took place, there were as many early outbreaks during both epidemics in rural areas as within large population centers. However, given the large pools of susceptibles within urban complexes, population sizes could be used to predict rates of increase *only after the epidemics were well underway.* The diffusion was not hierarchical in accordance with city size, and there was no direct linear correlation between national transportation routes and early outbreaks.

The recent re-emergence of H_1N_1, and its apparent co-mingling with H_3N_2, now offers an opportunity to determine whether similar patterns can be identified during the late 1970s and early 1980s. Research on this question is currently in progress.

Models of geographic spread

K. Choi

ABSTRACT

Influenza data are viewed longitudinally as the superposition of two stochastic processes. The first process generates the expected (non-epidemic) pneumonia and influenza (P & I) mortality for various locations. The second process is the superposition of two further stochastic processes: one of these is a two-dimensional (time-place) point process, the other is determined by the properties of the virus and the environment.

So far, we have only discussed the Russian model for the geographic spread of influenza epidemics, which is a deterministic mass-action model. I shall briefly describe an alternative approach, that of constructing a stochastic model for the temporal and geographic spread of epidemics.

The basic idea is to view the influenza data longitudinally as a superposition of two stochastic processes. The first process leads to the expected P & I mortality for various locations. A model for the process, such as a spatial ARIMA model (see Cliff and Ord, 1981) could be fitted to the non-epidemic adjusted data, as in the ARIMA model for the temporal spread of epidemics which was proposed by Choi and Thacker (1981). In such a model, the P & I mortality for each week is associated with each location (e.g., a city), and the current expected P & I mortality for a given location is expressed as a function of the past weekly mortality data in various locations.

The second process leads to outbreaks of influenza epidemics. This process, in turn, is the superposition of two further stochastic processes. The first of these is a two-dimensional (time-place) point process, i.e. the process which triggers an epidemic in various locations at different times, according to a probability which can be estimated from past data. Given that an epidemic is triggered, its course is described by the second stochastic process, which is determined by the characteristics of the virus and by environmental factors. The second process could be a stochastic analogue of a mass-action model.

We plan to analyze retrospectively the data from the 121-city P & I mortality surveillance system, using the above-mentioned approach.

References

Choi, K., and Thacker, S. B. (1981) An evaluation of influenza mortality surveillance, 1962-1979: (I) Time series forecasts of expected pneumonia and influenza deaths, (II) Percentage of pneumonia and influenza deaths as an indicator of influenza activity, *Amer. J. Epid.*, *113*, 3.

Cliff, A. D., and Ord, J. K. (1981) *Spatial processes, models and applications*, London: Prior/Methuen.

Session VI: Discussion of presentation by Pyle

Rapporteur: Spicer

J. Smith asked whether Pyle's method would indicate in advance areas in which special immunization programs might be useful.

Pyle replied that this might be possible, but only if based on a model of finer subdivision than an American state.

Tyrrell mentioned Sayers' work on the construction of contour maps of the spread of rabies. He wondered whether such methods would be feasible with influenza.

Bailey commented that Sayers' method was based on using the filtering techniques of communications engineering to eliminate noise, and should in principle be applicable.

Spicer said that such techniques might not be so effective in the rather erratic spread of influenza along paths of travel. He had heard that Sayers was applying his methods to data on influenza in London, but no results had yet been reported to his knowledge.

Stuart-Harris showed a slide of the spread of an H_1N_1 epidemic from a rural focus in Sardinia to northern Europe. He pointed out that identification of this spread had only been possible because there had been no recent H_1N_1 epidemic in the area due to the same subtype of virus.

J. Smith asked Haggett whether there was evidence of fade-out of influenza in Iceland.

Haggett thought that the disease was probably maintained in the more populous coastal regions around Reykjavik, where a study of monthly records since 1900 showed few non-reporting spells of more than a month or so since 1940. He was interested in Sayers' work, but did not think it was applicable to the discontinuous type of spread that occurred in Iceland.

Tyrrell suggested that spread from a center by "social" paths could perhaps be studied in the type of records kept by Dr Pickles, in Wensleydale, England.

L. Smith agreed, and suggested that it was equally important to identify contacts in which there was no subsequent infection.

Haggett said he had used multi-dimensional scaling methods to construct maps based on lags in infection times between areas, rather than on geographic distances. These gave a more informative picture of the progress of an epidemic.

Discussion of presentation by Choi

Spicer observed that Choi's approach required a definition of the word "epidemic".

Choi provided the following definition: 'A number of cases exceeding the normal number by 1.65 standard deviations, the "normal" number being derived from selected years of low incidence'.

J. Smith asked whether Choi had incorporated data on vaccination, and on deaths in people over 65 years of age, in his model.

Choi replied that he had not yet done so.

J. Smith, returning to Pyle's paper, asked whether the mode of spread in epidemic years was different from that for endemic influenza.

Pyle replied that spread in epidemic years was faster.

Spicer asked Choi whether he had considered using the Russian method of modelling spread between major cities.

Choi replied that he had, and would use a similar index of contacts between towns, based on the product of their populations.

Haggett suggested that the Russian type of model might involve attempts to estimate too many parameters, and that some economy could be obtained by defining sub-areas within larger geographic units.

Choi said he would economize as far as possible by selecting a subset of the total available cities.

Fine quoted Stuart-Harris as saying that the speed of spread of pandemics had not increased very much in the last 50 years, in relation to the speed of transport. He also quoted Bailey as saying that pandemics did not follow obvious paths of world travel. He asked for comments on these anomalies. He also mentioned that the Russians wished to extend their present epidemic model to the international level.

Stuart-Harris agreed that spread was surprisingly slow. He noted that, for example, Asian 'flu had spread quickly to Darwin, in northern Australia, where there was an epidemic, but did not then spread quickly along travel routes to the main population centers in the south and east of the country.

He felt that ships were a much more potent vehicle of spread than aircraft, and that spread usually required several cases to be introduced into the new population, although a single case had once been known to infect all the other passengers in an aircraft.

Haggett reported that, in Iceland, records suggested that local spread in small communities was usually initiated by a single case. He wondered whether the incease in tourism might introduce a type of passenger more likely to acquire and transmit infection.

Bailey remarked that the preliminary WHO study of pandemic spread had not enabled clear statements to be made about the patterns of spread observed.

Stuart-Harris suggested that viral spread might be better studied by a virologist knowing the natural history of the disease, than by a statistician.

Bailey said that viral characteristics were taken into account but there were anomalies, such as the failure of a new virus to enter an area while the older strain remained prevalent.

Stuart-Harris surmised that the new virus might be seeding itself by sub-clinical infection.

J. Smith noted that, when asked three years ago, the Russians did not think extension of their model to Europe was possible.

Choi pointed out, however, that the Russians had shown great willingness to collaborate with the USA.

Bailey did not think the Russians needed any help, but remarked that they were, nevertheless, very willing to collaborate in the area of systems analysis.

Abstract of discussion

1. Although there is a broad relationship between the spread of influenza and normal channels of communication, some anomalies exist. In particular, the speed of spread of the disease has increased very little since the current pattern of influenza epidemiology emerged in about 1890. The aeroplane may be a much less effective means of spread than the ship, which allows the maturation of a number of cases and consequently the arrival of a large dose of virus in a susceptible community. The expansion of tourism by air might, however, result in more rapid and profuse spread of the disease.

2. Another possible cause of the slow and sometimes anomalous spread of the disease is the fact that new antigenic types often take a year or two to establish themselves in a susceptible community, while giving rise to subclinical cases. Also, it is difficult to trace patterns of spread unless the type of antibodies in the spreader is different from the prevailing type in the community.

3. Haggett's studies in Iceland clearly showed person-to-person spread of infection, which in isolated rural communities often arose from a single immigrant. They also showed that the temporal spread of the virus was closely related to the times of travel between communities, as opposed to the geographic distances.

4. The Russian model of spread is probably not applicable to western European conditions, owing to the volume and rapidity of inter-city migration. However, Choi intends to try incorporating a travel factor in his surveillance system in the USA.

5. The methods introduced by Professor Sayers, of Imperial College, London, for studying the spread of rabies are based on methods of smoothing developed in communications engineering. There was some doubt as to whether they could be used for studying the behavior of influenza, particularly of the kind that Haggett observed in Iceland. It is understood that Sayers is, nevertheless, applying his methods to influenza in London.

6. Further studies of spread on a small scale, such as that of Dr Pickles in Wensleydale, could be useful.

Session VII

Intervention models and vaccine strategy

Elveback

J. Smith

Intervention models and vaccine strategy (1)

L. R. Elveback

ABSTRACT

If models of vaccination and other intervention measures are to have useful application to public health policy, they must be specific for the virus, the population structure, and the vaccine. In addition, they must be understandable by those who make policy decisions.

It is doubtful whether a single model can serve for all purposes. Operational models for public health decision-making should therefore be encouraged at the following levels:

1. The level of basic research, concerning the relative importance of various characteristics of the virus, the population, and the vaccine, which determine outcome in terms of the total number of cases of illness or some other objective function.

2. The national policy level. Here, the cost of operation of the model is not of great importance, since even the most detailed stochastic simulation models involve costs which are small in comparison to the implementation of immunization programs.

3. Implementation of national policy at the local level. Here, cost is important, as are the size and type of computer needed.

There are model properties which are important at all three levels:

1. The model should be sufficiently realistic to be understood both by policy-makers and by those who implement policy. This points to the need for education, not only about the behavior of influenza viruses and the limitations of the herd immunity approach, but also about the usefulness of modelling as an aid to decision-making.

2. The model should be agent-specific and, through appropriate changes in parameter values, be applicable to different influenza A viruses, such as the Asian and Hong Kong viruses and the expected H_4 virus.

3. The model should be specific to a given population and social structure, should allow for differences in vaccine strategy with differences

in age distribution, and should allow for other intervention methods, such as the closing of schools and the cancellation of indoor sports events.

4. The model should be vaccine-specific. Further information is urgently needed on the speed of response to, and the failure rate of, both inactivated and live virus vaccine. The model should provide information concerning the amount of lead time (before the virus reaches the local population) that is necessary in order for a vaccination campaign to be worthwhile. This point is illustrated in the figure.

5. A model which allows the optimal allocation of a limited supply of vaccine has a great advantage (Longini et al., 1978). For this purpose

Median epidemic size (number of infections) with vaccination of 70% of schoolchildren, as function of time of vaccination and type of vaccine

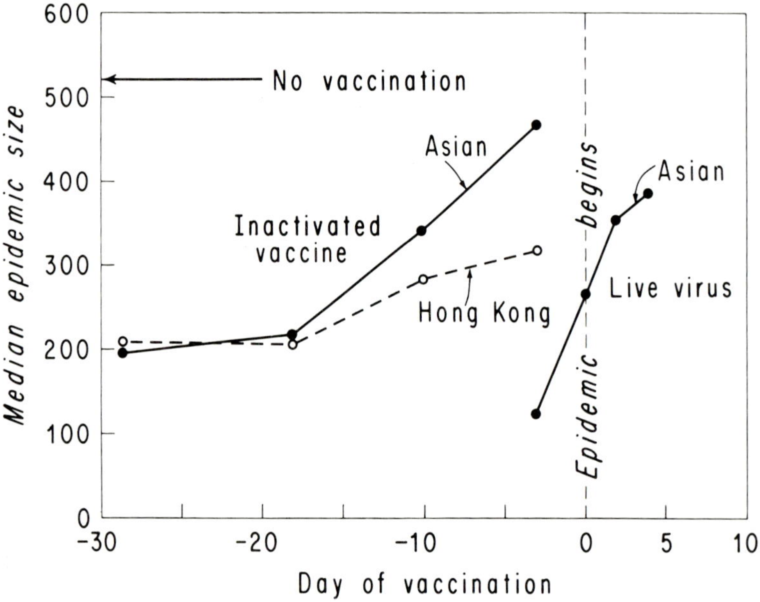

The time of vaccination had less effect on the size of the Hong Kong epidemics than of the Asian epidemics, as the former developed more slowly (with 28% of school cases in the first two weeks, as compared with 90% during the Asian epidemics). The right-hand curve shows the result of using a live virus vaccine, which has the advantage of interfering with the wild virus during the period needed for the development of specific immunity.

From Elveback et al. (1976).

the local age distribution and social structure, particularly for young adults, are very important.

6. In the optimization procedure, an appropriate objective function must be chosen. This involves difficulties in weighing immunization of individuals in high-risk groups, for their own protection, against immunization of those most instrumental in spreading infection, for the protection of the community.

7. While models which are appropriate for the local implementation of national policy are important, their usefulness will increase as they become appropriate for larger and larger areas.

References

Elveback, L. R. et al. (1976) An influenza simulation model for immunization studies, *Amer. J. Epid.*, *103*, 152-65.

Longini, I. M., Ackerman, E., and Elveback, L. R. (1978) An optimization model for Influenza A epidemics, *Math. Biosci.*, *38*, 141-57.

Intervention models and vaccine strategy (2)

J. W. G. Smith

ABSTRACT

Of various possibilities for intervention, vaccine is at present the only serious one. Current vaccination strategy is aimed primarily at high-risk groups. Vaccine effectiveness is uncertain, and may vary with the viral strain and the circumstances under which the vaccine is used. Pandemic vaccine probably requires two spaced injections in order to protect. The value of annual injections of updated inter-pandemic vaccines is uncertain.

It can be difficult to vaccinate target groups owing to social attitudes and logistic and financial obstacles. Intervention modelling should indicate the "most effective" targets for vaccination. It is necessary to establish whether a model based on outbreaks in one part of the world can be applied elsewhere, or whether different models are needed for different areas.

The value of modelling and intervention campaigns should be studied during the next pandemic, and the results applied to subsequent pandemics.

First, a reminder of current vaccination strategy. It is aimed primarily at high-risk groups, such as people with bronchitis, or the elderly in institutions, who are likely to die from an attack of influenza. The groups that are selected as this primary target may vary in different countries; in the USA, for example, they include people over the age of 65 years. I believe there is no solid evidence that a vaccination program aimed at these various high-risk groups produces the result that is hoped for, although it is entirely reasonable to give such groups a high priority for vaccination.

A second target group in many countries is those who are believed to have a high risk of becoming infected, such as health workers or residential schoolchildren. Although the degree of priority that should be given to offering vaccine to groups liable to high attack rates is arguable, it is nevertheless common practice.

A third category of target groups for vaccination depends on social criteria, which vary in different countries. Some countries might choose the armed forces, for example. In the USSR, vaccination is practiced widely in industry. In the UK, trade unions sometimes encourage and support vaccination; this does not form part of the national strategy, but is regarded by the unions as of possible benefit to their members. These offers of vaccination to various social groups are, however, based upon unproven expectations, rather than upon incontrovertible evidence that the vaccination program produces the required effect.

I should like also to remind you about the vaccine itself. As Dr Elveback pointed out, we are at present concerned with killed vaccine given by injection. There is reasonable evidence, based upon the results of controlled trials using a suitable placebo, that a single injection of an inter-pandemic vaccine will give about 70% immunity against natural challenge. However, the actual degree of protection may vary from year to year, depending on the vaccine and its relationship to the prevalent virus; thus a model may have to be virus-specific and vaccine-specific. There is, however, uncertainty about the results of annual injections of updated inter-pandemic vaccines, and I shall refer to this again later. For pandemic vaccines there is serological evidence, especially from intensive studies of the swine influenza vaccine, that two spaced injections are needed to stimulate an antibody level compatible with immunity. However, there are no natural challenge data to demonstrate the value of modern pandemic vaccines; there is a probability, but no certainty, that a pandemic vaccine can be protective, and this effect might differ depending upon whether the new virus possesses a new HA antigen only, or both a new HA and NA antigen.

The possibilities for intervention, which are well covered in Paul Fine's background paper, can be looked at conventionally in terms of the source of infection, the route by which it is transmitted, and the susceptible host. We can consider intervention at any of these points.

The source of influenza during an outbreak is presumably an infected person. The types of intervention which are available include isolation, quarantine, and chemotherapy, but there is no evidence that any of these have an effect on influenza epidemics.

As regards the route of transmission, the bulk of evidence suggests that this is airborne, probably mainly via droplets rather than by less efficient droplet nuclei. This implies that fairly close contact is important. Airborne infection might possibly be impeded by the wearing of masks, a common practice in China according to newspaper photographs. Again, I do not think there is any evidence that the practice is of value, although it might be if the masks are efficient. Treatment of the indoor air with ultra-violet light has been studied by a number of groups, mostly in relation to operating-theater infection but also in the control of airborne infection in schools. The general findings were that it had no measurable effect on infection transmitted by droplets, although it had some effect on measles in the British school studies. It is possible that adequate spacing of beds in institutions might have an effect if droplets are the main transmission route, and that avoidance of crowds during epidemics could help. But again, there appears to be no evidence of protection by such measures. The main effort, as we are all aware, must be directed towards raising the resistance of the susceptible individual.

The main procedure by which the resistance of the individual can be raised is prophylactic vaccination. There are other possibilities, such as chemoprophylaxis. Amantadine and other antiviral drugs may have a prophylactic effect against influenza, and could be used in combination with vaccination, for example in dealing with the threat of an epidemic in an old people's home. The use of chemoprophylaxis for 2-3 weeks, together with vaccination, might eliminate the critical period, which Dr Elveback has demonstrated, before immunization becomes effective. Passive immunization has also been used on a fairly large scale in the USSR, where supplies of normal human immunoglobulin are moved across the country according to the predictions of models, but I have not seen clear evidence that this has an effect. As Dr Elveback mentioned, control using live virus vaccine is a possibility, but the current availability of live vaccine is so limited that this is not a serious intervention possibility at the moment.

Figure 1 shows a real model of influenza, that of a virus particle. I'm fairly familiar with this kind of model, and it may be the best we can come up with by the end of the session!

Figure 2 shows the results of a study by Hoskins et al. (1979), which have cast doubt on the value of annual vaccination with updated inter-pandemic vaccine. The group concerned are boys in a boarding school in England, who were given either no vaccine or various combinations of different vaccines: Hong Kong vaccine at the beginning of the Hong Kong era, Hong Kong vaccine one year and Port Chalmers vaccine another year, or A/England vaccine. The figure shows that the total cumulative clinical attack rates over the years of the study were not very different in the different vaccinated groups, as compared with the boys who had no vaccine. This result is worrying. The study was on a relatively small scale, but it was carefully done. There is much interest in repeating this study, but it would now be very difficult to do so in England or the USA because of the problems of taking blood samples from schoolchildren once or twice a year, of securing volunteer groups to receive influenza vaccines, and of finance.

One aspect which Dr Elveback touched on, and which I find very interesting, is that, although a model might indicate who should be immunized, it may be very difficult to reach that target group, at least with

FIGURE 1

Three-dimensional model of the influenza virus

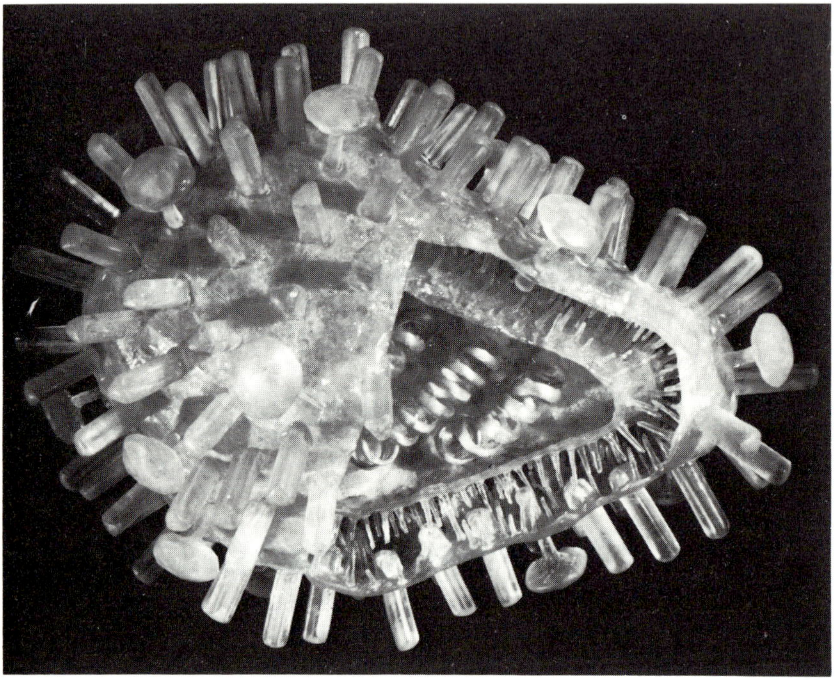

By courtesy of the British Science Museum.

influenza vaccine. Figure 3 shows the acceptance rate among different industrial groups who were offered vaccine in different years. These groups were vigorously pressed to accept vaccination, by means of campaigns which were strongly supported by the trade unions and management, and which involved posters and individual letters to all employees. In Group C, a factory of about 6,000 employees, the acceptance rate was 40% in the first year but fell to about 16% after four years of offering the vaccine each winter. Annual influenza vaccination campaigns tends, in my experience, to become less and less productive.

The pattern of acceptance among employees in the factory mentioned above is illustrated in Figure 4. The younger men, who perhaps could be an important target group, had a much lower acceptance rate than men aged 25-34 years, who were more likely to have families and financial responsibilities, and to be anxious to stay at work. The elderly, who could likewise be an important target group, were also relatively reluctant to accept vaccine. Married women accepted vaccine most readily, although in terms of industrial economy they might be a less important target than men. These difficulties of acceptance could seriously erode the effectiveness of a vaccination campaign. This is not to decry the value of identifying target groups by means of modelling, but we should be aware that achieving the targets set by a model may be very difficult. But perhaps an ideal model would also take these factors into account.

FIGURE 2

Cumulative clinical attack rates of influenza among 375 boys in a boarding school, during three outbreaks

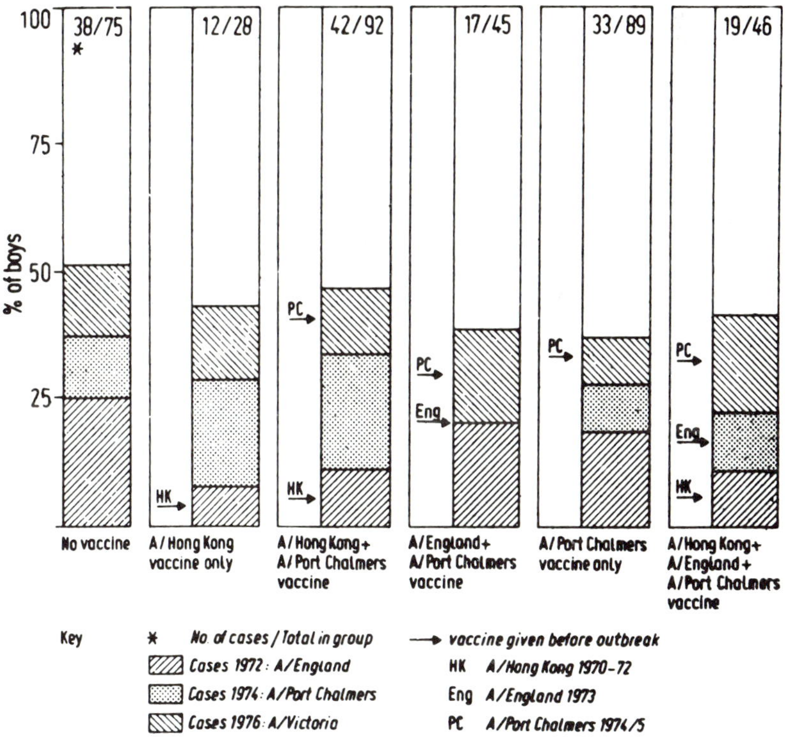

From Hoskins et al. (1979).

FIGURE 3

Influenza vaccine acceptance rates among different industrial groups offered vaccine in different years

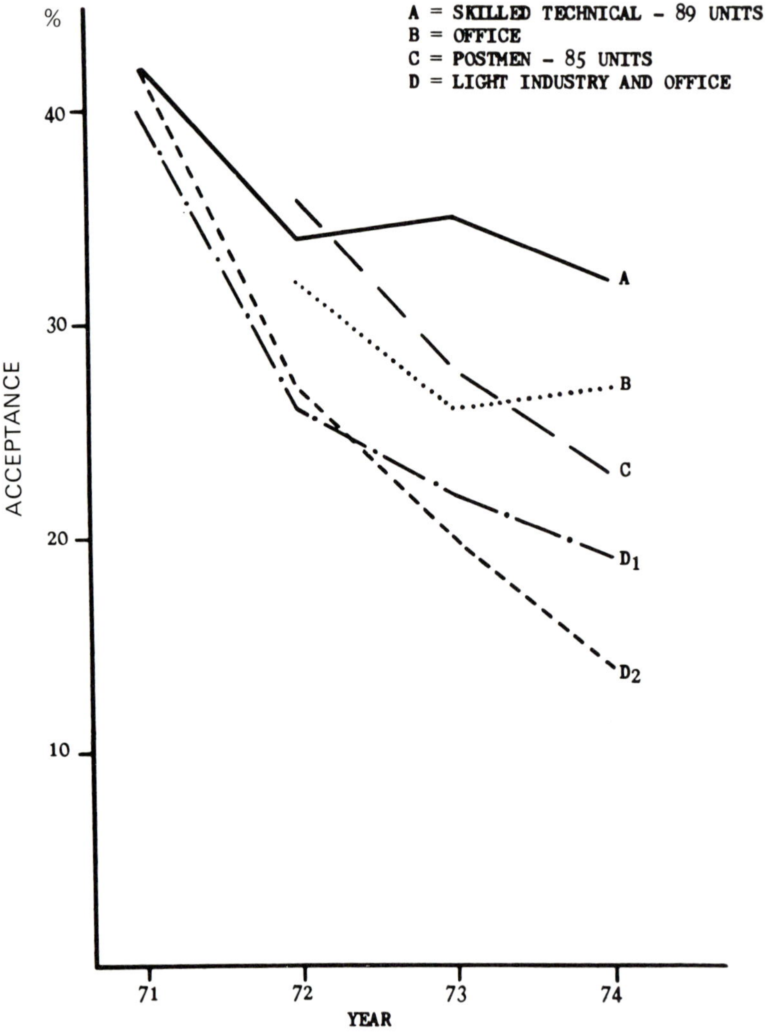

The reasons for not accepting vaccine are quite interesting. One reason is that even the most purified influenza vaccine does cause minor reactions which, although trivial, seem nevertheless to deter many people. Apathy is a strong factor, judging by the findings of a questionnaire survey among over 2,000 employees (Figure 5). A quarter of the respondents said they refused vaccine because they did not believe it to be effective, and this is understandable. In Europe, and probably in

FIGURE 4

Pattern of acceptance of influenza vaccine among factory employees

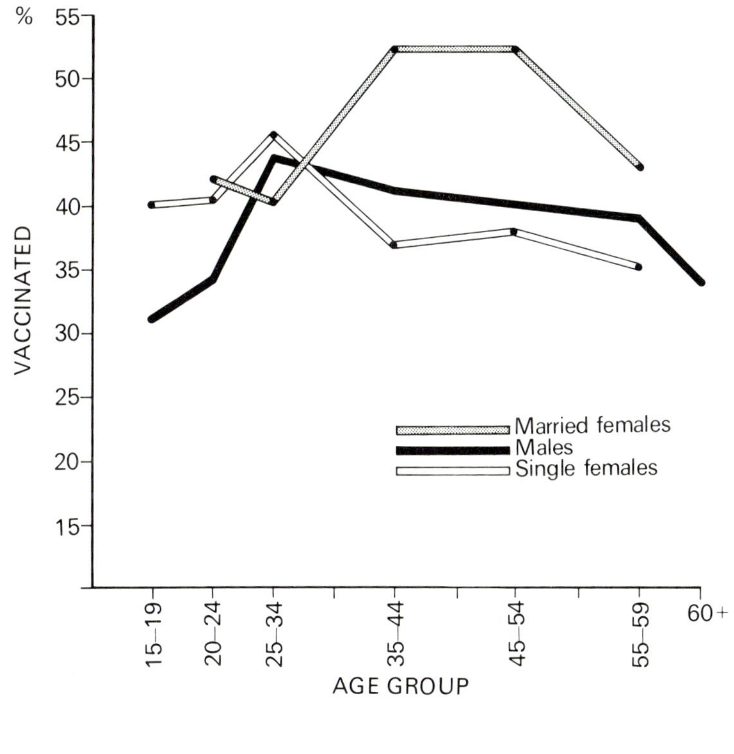

From Smith, J. W. G., Pollard, R., Fletcher, W. B., Barker, R., and Lewis, J. R. (1974) *Brit. J. Indust. Med., 31*, 292.

North America as well, both the lay public and practicing GPs tend to confuse influenza with other causes of upper respiratory infection, including colds. In an English winter, the average number of clinically apparent colds per person could be as many as four or five. Against this background "noise", the vaccinee is often unable to perceive any effect of influenza vaccine.

FIGURE 5

Reasons given for refusing influenza vaccine, by 2,290 employees in factories in which vaccine was also offered in the previous year

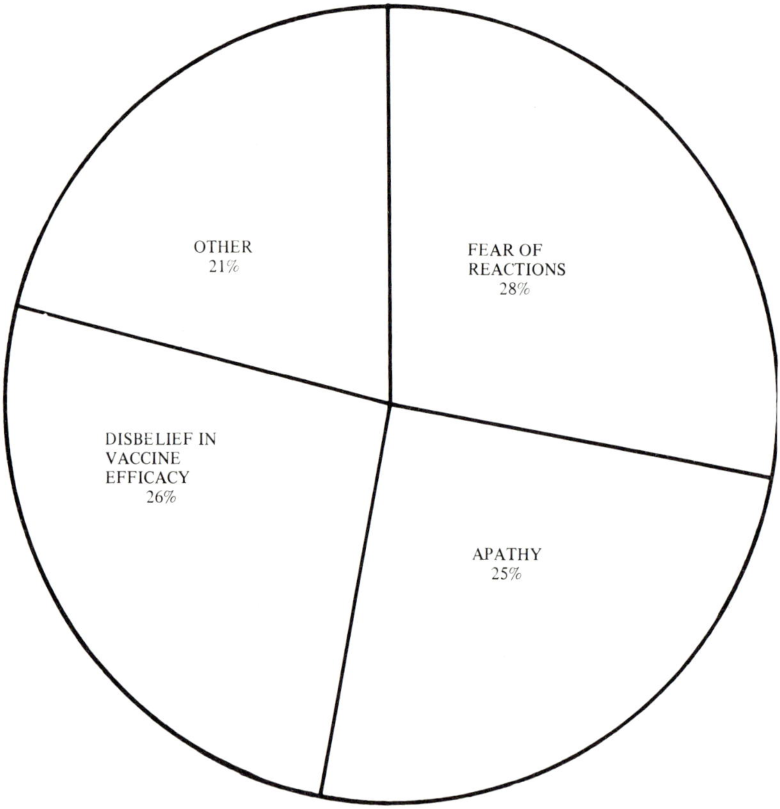
OTHER
21%
FEAR OF
REACTIONS
28%
DISBELIEF IN
VACCINE
EFFICACY
26%
APATHY
25%

An important practical limitation to vaccination is the short period that is available for manufacture of vaccine, particularly in a pandemic year. This implies that there may be only limited vaccine supplies, and only a short period of time available for its administration. Great achievements are possible, as in the swine influenza vaccine program, in which about 40 million immunizations were carried out within a period of about three months. But it would be very difficult to implement another vaccination program on such a large scale, in view of the poor history of that event.

Two other questions affecting vaccination strategy have to be offset against the potential benefits: cost (influenza vaccine is not cheap) and side-effects. Although most side-effects are not very significant, a study in the Post Office Giro factory showed that reactions nevertheless gave rise to about 2.8 days of absence per hundred vaccinated employees. This factor has to be taken into account, as well as more serious effects such as neurological complications.

To consider finally the field I have come to this meeting to learn about: intervention models. Modelling has to be based at present on the use of vaccine rather than any other intervention technique. At a practical level, I would first like to know: Can models indicate the "most effective" targets? I put "most effective" in inverted commas, because to define the target is only partly a medical or scientific problem; it is also a social and political decision. Society has to decide, for example, whether it is more important to reduce deaths in old age or to keep the factories going. An ideal model should show the potential impact of a vaccination campaign on each of these and other targets, so that health administrators can reach an appropriate decision on their own terms.

A second important point for intervention modelling is whether experience in one part of the world can be used to optimize vaccine use elsewhere. If the results of an intervention program could be monitored in one part of the world and then reliably be applied elsewhere, this would be a practical advance. There is scope for preliminary work here, to establish whether the parameters of an outbreak caused by a particular virus in one part of the world differ greatly from those in another part of the world, and whether any differences can be explained, for example by social or other factors. If this is not possible we are in great difficulty, because a different model would then need to be prepared for every sort of society and geographic area.

The third point of potential practical importance is the extent to which experience in one pandemic can be related to future pandemics. I suspect that the characteristics of a pandemic virus (that is, a virulent virus attacking a population without HA and, possibly, NA antibodies) are much more important than environmental factors in determining the severity of its effect. Consequently, if we were to make studies directed towards the use of modelling in divising vaccination strategy in a forthcoming pandemic, it is likely that those results could be applied to later pandemics. A vigorous program to study the value of modelling in planning intervention campaigns in the next pandemic therefore seems to be justified. We may not succeed in reducing the impact of the pandemic, but the results could be of great value in dealing with succeeding pandemics.

Reference

Hoskins, T. W., Davis, J. R., Smith, A. J., Miller, C. L., and Allchin, A. (1979) *Lancet, i,* 33.

Session VII: Discussion of presentations by Elveback and J. Smith

Rapporteur: Haggett

Public health workers would find great value in a model which had been sufficiently well validated to enable the investigation or prediction of the benefits, and other consequences, of a wide range of intervention strategies.

Stuart-Harris believed that the most basic need is to develop models which will contribute to solving the practical problem of stopping an epidemic, for example through simulating the likely effects of different vaccination strategies. They might help to answer the following questions: What vaccination rate is needed to protect a population against a virus with given characteristics? Which groups within a population should be protected first? What is the likely impact on the spread of influenza of vaccinating particular age groups, e.g. schoolchildren? We might learn from the Japanese experience of regular programs for the immunization of schoolchildren. A model should be able to help in deciding between options, for example when there is a shortage of vaccine or money, or where there might be a long-term danger of reduced acceptance rate of vaccination if it were made available too frequently in non-critical years.

Elveback pointed out the cost implications of computer models. Both her own model and that of Longini needed a sufficient number of individuals in each status group for spread to be considered as a continuous rather than a discrete process. Experience with a population of 2,000 suggested that extension to larger populations would bring major cost increases.

Choi and J. Smith raised the question of the appropriate decision-making level to which any model must relate. In the USA, the state is probably the critical level for decisions on vaccination policy, while decision-making at the lower, county level has less effect. On the other hand, action at the local level is essential in ensuring that vaccines are available for distribution, and in ensuring that information is made available to clinics, physicians, and the general public.

Elveback cited experience in the USA which suggests that suitably structured committees, and the involvement of public health nurses, can considerably increase the vaccination acceptance rate at the local level. The local county also provides the demographic statistics needed for model calibration.

Fine and Spicer considered that the mathematical structure of epidemiological models will be important in determining their suitability for local use. In general, any model which is stochastic and which needs random-number generation will be costlier in computer time. Deterministic models (including the Russian model) are likely to be easier to use locally, but local parameters will need to be estimated. A federal or national center could play an important role in making software available locally, or in making estimates on behalf of local authorities.

Bailey questioned the need for different models for different epidemiological situations. There might be a case for models which are strain-specific, or which differentiate between endemic and epidemic periods. But existing models can generally be structured more effectively, so as to incorporate parameters which can cope with these variations. There is a need to move on from models which replicate an empidemiological process to those which relate to problems of resource allocation. We shall then need to clarify the objectives of any intervention policy. For example, are we interested in maximizing the number of disease-free people, in protecting certain high-risk groups, or in minimizing costs due to absenteeism from work?

Elveback pointed out that the Longini model uses two objective functions, based on (a) the number of years of life lost and (b) the cost of working days lost. She recalled that one economist, Kavet, had put the direct and indirect costs of the 1968-70 influenza epidemic in the USA at about $5 billion.

Stuart-Harris drew a distinction between the modelling of major pandemics and of more localized outbreaks. In pandemics, antibodies are more prevalent in a population once the main wave has gone through, by which time there is not much opportunity for vaccination seriously to modify the attack rate. Thus, while protection rates of 40-70% can be obtained in inter-pandemic periods, they are much lower during pandemics. The efficacy of a vaccine can be measured either in terms of antibody levels or of protection against illness; in his view, only the former measure is effective.

Fine noted that vaccine efficacy is conventionally expressed by the following term:

$$\text{vaccine efficacy} = \frac{AR_{NV} - AR_{V}}{AR_{NV}}$$

where AR is the attack rate, and NV and V refer to non-vaccinated and vaccinated populations, respectively. Here, a tendency for higher attack rates among non-vaccinated persons may in theory be reduced to some degree because of the indirect protective effect of herd immunity; but it is not known what proportion of a population needs to be vaccinated in order to achieve such "herd immunity". This will in any case be affected by the degree of closeness of the population, in terms of its geographic pattern of contacts.

Several participants commented on the difficulty of using vaccination data. *Tyrrell* observed that killed virus under the skin had a different impact on antibody production than live virus in the respiratory tract. More work is needed to compare placebos with vaccines administered at different lengths of time before an outbreak. *J. Smith* confirmed the difficulty of drawing inferences from vaccination observations. He cited studies which indicated that, although higher influenza attack rates occurred in people who were unvaccinated as compared with those who were vaccinated, the previous illness history also showed significant differences between the two groups; those who accepted vaccination were, in these studies, among the healthier section of the sampled population.

Stuart-Harris described the differences in the rate of increase in mortality, during the first few weeks of major influenza epidemics in England and Wales. The evidence from the work of Logan and MacKay (1951) is that the rate of increase varies significantly. Vaccination seems to give no protection when there is an antigenic shift in the virus, but antigenic drift can be coped with by vaccination and other protective measures. The question is whether widespread vaccination campaigns should be attempted during inter-pandemic periods, since the acceptance rate of vaccination might well increase if campaigns are less frequent.

In discussion, it was clear that the acceptance rate of vaccination is highly variable. Old people were cited as an example of a high-risk group with a low acceptance rate. They have a rather strong resistance to the idea of being vaccinated, while physicians have mixed views as to the usefulness of any general program for this group. The case of schoolchildren is perhaps easier, in view of their role as virus-spreaders within the population. Even where vaccine is given, evidence was cited of very different levels of protection from the different vaccines available, and of cross-protection between immunizations.

The problems encountered in increasing the acceptance rate of vaccination brought the discussion back to the group's initial concern for effective intervention models. *Bailey* drew comparisons with a typhoid model, in which conclusions about endemic levels were sensitive to only four out of 25 parameters. Field application of models might be aided by stripping down some existing models into a simpler and more robust form. *J. Smith* concluded that this would lead to the need for more accurate estimations of the really critical parameters. *Bailey* also drew a distinction between those models which represent an epidemiological process, and those which help directly in decision-making. In malaria control, for example, there is a need to decide how much of scarce resources should be spent on killing mosquitoes, and how much on getting drugs to people. Decisions may depend on specifying carefully the objectives of a health program. For example, work is being done at IIASA (International Institute of Applied Systems Analysis), in Vienna, to explore "inferred value" models of intervention and health care, in which estimates are made of the values administrators appear to be applying in deciding priorities. Once these values are clarified, we may wish to confirm or reject them. The construction of effective intervention models might need to draw on a wider range of disciplines than has commonly been involved in epidemiological studies in the past.

Reference

Logan, W. P. D., and MacKay, D. G. (1951) Development of influenza epidemics, *Lancet, i*, 284-5.

Abstract of discussion

1. Technical solutions are needed in order to modify existing models so that they can be used by local public health authorities with limited resources.

2. Attempts to optimize a vaccination strategy must depend on an intervention policy with clear short-term and long-term objectives.

Session VIII

Recommendations

Recommendations

Rapporteurs: Fine and Tyrrell

A. Further studies of the patterns of spread of epidemics

1. Special data sources, such as school absenteeism records, should be examined in order to study the pattern of spread of influenza.

2. Excess mortality approaches should be applied to specific disease conditions associated with increased mortality risks during influenza epidemics.

3. Available data on past pandemics should be examined in order to see how predictable their course was in retrospect. In particular, the shape of epidemics in the early phases of these pandemics should be compared with patterns recorded later in their course. To what extent do the transmission parameter λ and the basic reproduction rate α of a shift virus remain constant, in different parts of the world at different times during the pandemic?

B. Further studies of existing models

1. The sensitivity of the Russian model to changes in the $\lambda S_0 = \alpha_0$ parameter should be explored.

2. An effort should be made to reduce both the Russian and Elveback-Longini models so that they can be run on a minicomputer. The structural analogies between these models should be explored, on the hypothesis that they are basically the same model. So far, their similarities have been overlooked.

3. Longini's deterministic analogue of the Elveback model should be written in a generally usable, machine-transferable form, possibly one which can be used where only minicomputers are available, and made available to researchers.

4. Modelling approaches analogous to those of Bartlett and of Yorke and Nathanson, on measles, should be applied to influenza, in order to investigate conditions for the maintenance of influenza virus in human populations.

5. Analyses of influenza trends should be carried out using models of the mass-action type and appropriate sero-epidemiological data. This will require longitudinal serological studies to be organized in a suitable population.

6. An effort should be made to study influenza in a small community, in the context of an Elveback-type, highly structured model.

C. Empirical studies to uncover additional factors which might be included in the further development of existing models

1. The influenza reports of RCGP spotter-practices should be examined, broken down by separate practices. They should be investigated in the context of local weather conditions, e.g. inversions, to see if weather factors trigger epidemics.

2. Changes in the transmission of influenza with season should be studied, as has been done for measles.

3. More work is needed, like that done in Iceland, to examine critically the data on movements and social contacts in relation to the spread of an epidemic in space and time. The unique records available in Iceland should be examined, to see whether they reveal the micro-ecology of influenza as clearly as they do that of measles.

4. The reasons why different cities or areas manifest different influenza epidemic patterns should be explored.

5. Statistics on population movements at the national and international levels should be examined, both currently and historically, in order to explore their implications for influenza spread.

D. Studies of the transmission coefficient λ and the number of susceptibles S_0

1. Serious studies should be made to apply mass-action models to available data, and to investigate whether λ, the transmission coefficient, and S_0, the number of susceptibles in a population, can be calculated theoretically and then related to, or deduced from, observations in the real world.

2. Thus far, all models of influenza have assumed a constant "transmission parameter" over time, during any epidemic. This may be erroneous. An attempt should be made to estimate the value of this parameter and its changes with time, weather, and antigenic drift or shift. For example, Choi proposes to use national US statistics to study λ as a function of time, weather, and antigenic drift, and to compare cities with high and low disease rates.

3. Efforts should be made to estimate the number of susceptibles at the start of an epidemic (S_0) by different means, both sero-epidemiological and theoretical. For example, it is recommended that someone look at data obtained from serological survey and RCGP records in the UK.

4. Similar studies should be done at an even more detailed level, possibly using the discrete Elveback model, from family studies such as outbreaks in residential schools, or the Virus Watch, or the Tecumseh or Wembley studies. The differences in spread in the young and old might be studied using data from periods when H_1N_1 and H_3N_2 are circulating. It might be desirable to set up further special studies which could be "switched on" when an epidemic threatened.

5. Laboratory-measurable properties of influenza viruses, e.g. virus excretion, stability to heat and drying, and infectivity, should be studied with the aim of relating these properties to transmissibility as described in epidemiological models, and to estimates of λ in the epidemics in which they were detected.

E. Further studies of the practical application of existing models (even though these are not fully validated)

1. Can one estimate λ and S_0, and hence the further behavior of an epidemic, from data collected in the first weeks?

2. What are likely to be the relative merits of public health measures, such as using inactivated or live vaccines, or chemotherapy, or closing schools?

3. Can we define the most effective mode of giving vaccine within a population to achieve different objectives, such as to reduce spread, incidence, or mortality, or calculate the influences on production or cost-effectiveness?

4. Further studies are required on the protective efficacy of influenza vaccines. An effort should be made to correlate seroconversion rates with protection of vaccinees against infection and/or disease.

5. Intervention models, such as those of Elveback and Longini, should be programmed to explore the effectiveness of chemoprophylaxis.

6. An operational research approach is needed, starting with a close study of what health administrators really need to know, and when, in order to make good decisions, e.g. the expected size of the epidemic and the number of cases needing hospital care.

F. Efforts to stimulate and support further work in this area

1. The Sandoz Institute has translated a booklet describing the Russian influenza modelling work. Similarly, the major monograph on this work is being translated by CDC. These translations should be made available to interested workers.

2. Interest in the subject should be stimulated by speedy publication of the background paper by Paul Fine and the summarized proceedings of this workshop.

3. Efforts should be made to ensure that all good proposals receive the support they need in the way of personal cooperation, the supply of data and, if necessary, finance.

4. A similar workshop should be convened in two or three years' time, for a detailed examination of the results which will have emerged by then.

Participants

Participants

Dr Norman BAILEY	chief, health statistical methodology, World Health Organization, Geneva
Dr Keewhan CHOI	mathematical statistician, consolidated surveillance and communications activity, bureau of epidemiology, Centers for Disease Control, Atlanta, Georgia, USA
Dr Lila ELVEBACK	professor of biostatistics, Mayo Medical School, Rochester, Minnesota, USA
Dr Paul FINE	lecturer in tropical hygiene, Ross Institute, London School of Hygiene and Tropical Medicine
Mr Adrian GRIFFITHS	head, health management and economics, Sandoz Institute, Geneva
Dr Peter HAGGETT	professor, department of geography, University of Bristol, UK
Dr Gerald PYLE	professor, department of geography and earth science, university of North Carolina, Charlotte, N.C., USA
Dr Philip SELBY	head, community medicine and epidemiology, Sandoz Institute, Geneva
Dr Joseph SMITH	director, National Institute for Biological Standards and Control, London
Mr Lionel SMITH	former president, commission for agricultural meteorology, World Meteorological Organization
Dr Clive SPICER	department of mathematical statistics and operational research, University of Exeter, UK
Sir Charles STUART-HARRIS	professor, department of virology, University of Sheffield, UK
Dr David TYRRELL	head, division of communicable diseases, and deputy director, clinical research center, Northwick Park Hospital, Harrow, Middlesex, UK

Observers

Dr Helmut BACHMAYER	department of immunobiology, Sandoz Research Institute, Vienna
Dr Mirko MAJER	head, immunobiology, Sandoz AG, Nuremberg